Natural Cures®

Secrets "They" Don't Want
You to Know About

New & Updated for 2015

Natural Cures®

Secrets "They" Don't Want
You to Know About

New & Updated for 2015

Kevin Trudeau

Natural Cures® Secrets "They" Don't Want You to Know About
New & Updated for 2015

This edition published by Natural Press, LLC
For information, address:

Natural Press, LLC
PO Box 8568
Pueblo, CO 81001

ISBN 13: 978-0-9911782-4-7

Interior design: The Printed Page, Phoenix, AZ

Manufactured in the United States of America

10 9 8 7 6 5 4 3 2 1

First Version

Contents

DISCLAIMER

You must know that everything I say in this book is simply my opinion and that there are many people who vehemently disagree with my conclusions. If you do anything I recommend without the supervision of a licensed medical doctor, it is at your own risk. The publisher, the author, the distributors and bookstores, present this information for educational purposes only. I am not making an attempt to prescribe any medical treatment, since under the laws of the United States only a licensed medical doctor (an MD) can do so. (How sad!)

This book contains only my opinions, thoughts, and conclusions. Again, it is for educational purposes only and you and only you are responsible if you choose to do anything based on what you read.

Kevin Trudeau

Acknowledgments

I would like to acknowledge the many people around the world who helped make this book and this mission possible. I can't name you all, but you know who you are. It's an honor to serve with you on this noble mission to educate the world about the evils of greed and the benefits of using natural methods to prevent and cure disease.

Ironically, I'd also like to thank the Federal Trade Commission and the Food and Drug Administration. Both agencies have inspired me to write this book, much like Goliath inspired David; and like David, with my measly slingshot I vow to help stop the needless suffering that their corruption has caused millions of people around the world.

Read This First

I congratulate you for having the courage to read this book. Your interest tells me that you're either sick and looking for natural cures, or you're worried about getting sick. You may also be concerned about the health and wellbeing of your family and friends. In order to get the most benefit from the information presented here, it's imperative that you read the book from start to finish. Don't jump ahead, or jump around the book looking for an immediate answer to a health related question. This applies to those of you who've seen my infomercial and may want the answer to a specific illness mentioned in the program. All of the information is presented in a specific order for a reason. Please be assured that if you start at the beginning and read the book in its entirety, by the time you reach the end you'll have a better understanding of the cause of your disease and you'll know that there is a natural cure for it. You'll also know what steps to take in order to cure yourself and remain healthy for life without drugs and surgery.

Please note that there are many important concepts discussed within these pages. Because these concepts are an important foundation to everything else that I discuss, in many instances I repeat them. This is done purposely, because in order for you to benefit from this information you must absolutely know, backwards and forwards, the basic foundational principles.

So let's begin the journey, and when you reach the end of this book I promise you, you'll never be the same!

Yours in health,

Kevin Trudeau

Introduction

Bill Gates was interviewed on The Larry King Show and when asked about his incredible wealth and success, he said "Larry, I was at the right place at the right time, and luck has a lot to do with that."

I believe that by reading this book, you are at the right place at the right time, right now. Maybe luck has something to do with it.

Bill continued, "But Larry, there were a lot of people at the same place I was. One difference was I had vision. I saw the potential that was there. And I took massive and immediate action."

Folks, as you read this book, will you see the potential that utilizing this information can have on your own health and wellbeing? Do you have the vision that you can prevent and cure almost all illness and disease with natural methods, without drugs, and without surgery? And will you take massive and immediate action by implementing the recommendations? If you do, you will succeed in your quest for longevity, health, and vitality.

There are natural cures for virtually every disease. The drug companies, the government, and a host of other organizations do not want you to know what these natural cures are. This book will give them to you. Since I first published it, I've received tens of thousands of letters and emails from people all around the world telling me how utilizing the information I've shared has changed their lives for the better. I hope it will have a positive impact on your life as well.

You'll be learning some new and exciting things here. The concepts are logical, easy to understand, and filled with common sense. However, the conclusions go against conventional wisdom. For you to fully grasp this information it's important that you ask yourself now just how "teachable" you are.

There is, in fact, a "teachability index," which will determine how easy learning new concepts will be for you. This teachability index consists of two variables. First, is your willingness to learn. Since you purchased this book, and you're taking the time to read it, on a scale of one to ten, you probably have a pretty high willingness to learn. However, the second variable is your willingness to accept change. If you're a ten on willingness to learn, but a zero on willingness to accept change, ten times zero is zero; therefore, your teachability index is nonexistent.

You must have a high willingness to accept change in order to fully grasp these concepts and benefit from them. I sincerely hope that you have a high teachability index.

As you read, please consider another important component to fully implementing the information in your daily life. Information is only useful when it is used. It can only be used when it's fully internalized; when you don't have to "think about it."

The four stages one goes through when learning any new information are:

1. Unconscious incompetence—this is the stage where you don't know that you don't know.

2. Conscious incompetence—this is the stage where you know you don't know.

3. Conscious competence—this is when you know that you know, but you have to consciously think about it.

4. Unconscious competence—this is when it's second nature; when the information is part of you and you know it as intrinsically as you know your own name; it's fully internalized and automatic.

When you read this book you'll go through the first three stages. When you finish, you'll have to implement the information for a time before reaching level four. When you do, you will quite possibly live a life that's healthy and disease free. You might even be fortunate enough to never get sick again. That may sound ambitious, but it is a real possibility. If you're ready, let the journey begin.

I Should Be Dead By Now

I was driving down the Tri-State Highway outside of Chicago, Illinois, in my brand new Corvette enjoying a beautiful sunny day. Suddenly I felt an enormous ripping pain in my chest. I could barely breathe; the pain was excruciating. I immediately pulled off to the side of the road. My life virtually flashed before my eyes and I thought, "Oh my God I'm having a heart attack and I'm only twenty-one years old!"

Just as quickly as the pain came, it vanished. I was left disoriented, and in a state of shock about what had just happened. I looked down at my new car phone, (yes, in the good old days before cell phones). I picked it up, called my secretary, and said, "I think I just had a heart attack."

Luckily within a few moments I felt fine. I figured that if it was a heart attack, it most likely didn't cause any major damage. But something was obviously wrong.

Over the next week I was examined by three of the top heart specialists in America. Through the use of the most advanced medical diagnostic devices, I learned that I had been born with a deformed heart; a severe mitral valve prolapse that would cause me major problems for the rest of my life. There was no cure.

> Skeptical, yet open to new ideas…What did I have to lose?

These top medical minds recommended experimental drugs, or risky surgery, both of which I was told had little promise. My life expectancy was to be very short.

I struggled to come up with an effective plan that could solve my medical dilemma. I was twenty-one years old with my whole life in front of me. I had to do something!

Months earlier I'd attended a lecture wherein I heard about a Harvard medical doctor named Yiwen Y. Tang, founder of the Century Clinic in Reno, Nevada. (Today the clinic is called Sierra Integrative Medical Center.) This MD, who'd been a MASH surgeon during the Korean War, had decided that standard medical procedures—drugs and surgery were not the best way to cure and prevent diseases. Instead, he was using a diagnostic device developed in Germany by Dr. Reinhold Voll called the Dermatron machine. Allegedly, in a matter of minutes, it could diagnose a person's medical problems. When the diagnosis was complete, homeopathic remedies were given to correct the imbalances and reverse and cure the disease.

At the time it sounded like hocus pocus. The words homeostasis, holistic healing, homeopathic remedies, acupuncture meridians, energy frequencies, imbalances, and the like were used in the lecture, replacing the standard vernacular that I knew: germs, bacteria, viruses, drugs, surgery, and genetics. Skeptical, yet open to new ideas, I flew to Reno to meet Dr. Tang. What did I have to lose?

Upon my arrival, the doctor asked me why I was there. Most of his patients were old and had severe medical problems. I, on the other hand, appeared to be healthy, and young, so he was puzzled by my desire for a diagnosis. I wanted to see if this Dermatron machine was legitimate, so I simply said, "I feel great. I just want a basic checkup."

He tested me with his magic machine and within two minutes the probe touched my heart meridian and registered very low energy. Dr. Tang looked at me with concern and said, "Son you have a heart problem." I was shocked by how quickly the diagnosis came. He just as quickly said, "Let me find out where it is."

He touched other meridian points. When he got to the mitral valve, once again, the machine registered very low energy. He looked at me and said matter-of-factly, "You have a mitral valve prolapse."

Needless to say, I was impressed. The medical doctors took days of testing to diagnose my mitral valve prolapse. This "energy machine" diagnosed it within minutes. I looked at Dr. Tang and said, "Yes I know, and I understand it's incurable." His response startled me. "In America it's incurable, but there are natural treatments in other countries that can reverse this problem in a matter of weeks. Unfortunately the FDA has not approved these treatments. So, yes, in America it is incurable."

He went on to explain a procedure of live cell injections that was available in Switzerland, or Mexico, but not accessible via legal treatment in the United States. The procedure would correct the problem by rebuilding the heart, ensuring that it would never return. I couldn't believe my ears. Effective natural treatments that are not approved by the FDA? Impossible!

This happened over twenty years ago. The treatment was inexpensive, all natural, painless, quick, and it *worked*. And to this day, that therapy is still illegal in America.

The most amazing part of this story is, after I received the natural treatment that was forbidden in America, I went back to the medical doctors who originally diagnosed my heart problem and asked to be tested again. My request was met with indignation. I was told that being tested again was a waste of time and money because it was impossible for the condition to change in two months. I demanded that they retest me anyway. The doctors humored me and they were stunned to find that I no longer had a mitral valve prolapse.

I was so excited to share how my problem had been cured. I thought certainly these doctors would want to know about an all natural treatment that could cure the incurable. Imagine my shock when I was told that the treatment could not have cured my disease but, rather, I must have been misdiagnosed in the first place. They tried to tell me that I never actually had the condition.

I couldn't believe my ears. These medical doctors would not accept the facts: I had a severe mitral valve prolapse—the pictures confirmed it; and then I no longer had a mitral valve prolapse—the pictures confirmed that, too.

I began to think of all of the people who would come to these medical doctors only to be told the bold-faced lie that their condition was incurable and could only be treated with drugs and surgery. Knowing that the established medical community would deny the existence of natural cures, and allow millions of people to suffer, and in many cases die, absolutely enraged me.

That event set in motion my lifelong mission of searching for natural remedies that don't include drugs or surgery, and natural treatments that prevent and cure illness and disease. It also exposed me to the organizations, companies, and government agencies that do not want you to know about these cures.

Today I live a full, healthy, and dynamic life. I don't take any drugs and I've had no surgeries. I haven't had a prescription or nonprescription drug in over twenty years. I virtually never get sick. Colds, flu, and all illnesses seem to pass me by. I've had numerous blood tests and other diagnostic tests every few years, just to make sure everything is within the normal range. The medical professionals who've examined and reviewed these results are amazed at the level of health that I enjoy. Am I lucky? Is it just genetics? Or are there some specific things that one can do to have a disease and illness-free life and enjoy vibrant health? Is it possible for you to go week after week, year after year, and never get sick? I strongly believe the answer is yes. This book specifically outlines the following things:

- ✔ Yes, there are all natural non-drug and nonsurgical cures for most every illness and disease.

- ✔ Yes, there are organizations, government agencies, companies and entire industries that are spending billions of dollars trying to hide these natural cures from you.

- ✔ Yes, every single nonprescription and prescription drug has adverse side effects and should virtually never be taken (with exceptions that I'll explain later).

It's important to note that I'm oversimplifying things in this book. That's because I'm not writing it for the medical community, scientists, researchers, or MDs. They're not going to agree with anything I say anyway. I'm writing this in plain English so that you can understand it.

Medical science always presents things as fact when actually it's opinion, based on information they have at the time. Throughout history, medical "facts" have been disproved time and time again.

The medical industry presents itself as the only source of truth when it comes to health, illness, and disease. They use words like "credible scientific evidence," "scientifically tested," and "scientifically proven." But what they're really presenting are theories, and theories change constantly. Here are examples of "medical facts" that have been proven wrong:

- ✔ Bloodletting was once proven to cure most illnesses. Now it is considered totally ineffective.

- ✔ Margarine was considered healthier than butter. Now research suggests that the opposite is true.

- ✔ Eggs were considered bad because of high cholesterol. Now research suggests that they aren't bad at all, they're actually healthy.

- ✔ Alcohol in all forms was said to be unhealthy and therefore should not be consumed. Then the medical community said that red wine was actually healthy for the heart, but other forms of alcohol were not. Now "medical science" says that all alcohol in moderation has health benefits.

- ✔ Chocolate and oily foods were touted to be a cause of acne. Now research suggests that they don't contribute to acne.

- ✔ Coffee was thought to be unhealthy. Now it's been discovered that coffee is a major source of antioxidants as well as a protective against liver cancer.

- ✔ Coconut oil was believed to be an unhealthy saturated fat. Now science says that coconut oil does not have a negative effect on cholesterol and is in fact good for the heart.

- ✔ Homosexuality was once classified as a disease.

✔ Medical doctors claimed that baby formula was much better than breast milk for children. Now the exact opposite is shown to be true.

✔ Milk was recommended for coating the stomach and alleviating stomach ulcers. Now it's discouraged and has been found to aggravate ulcers.

✔ Medical science at one time stated that diet had no effect on disease or illness. Now we're told that diet has a huge effect on the prevention and cause of disease.

✔ Medical science once had evidence that removing the tonsils and the appendix improved health and should be done to virtually everyone. Now the medical community has reversed that theory.

✔ Children with asthma were told to stay in enclosed pool areas because the humidity was good for their condition. Now research suggests that the chlorine in the air from pools actually makes asthma worse.

✔ The most obvious example of all is the fact that there are thousands of drugs that have been approved by the FDA because they were scientifically proven to cure, or prevent disease, and they were found to be safe to use. Then, years later, they've been taken off the market because they either did not cure or prevent those diseases, or the side effects were so adverse that they're too dangerous to use.

It saddens me when I see doctors on TV stating things as *fact* when they should be qualifying their comments with such phrases as: "it appears," "based on the current research we have," "it seems that," or "we believe this to be true, however, we also know that as more research and observations are evaluated this may change in the future."

This is not happening. Medical doctors are still looked upon as gods. Whatever they say is taken as absolutely true. No one else can say anything about health, illness, or disease with the credibility of a medical doctor. In my opinion, that's just wrong. Medical doctors are trained to prescribe drugs, or cut out parts of a person's anatomy (surgery). They aren't trained in preventing disease and, most importantly, they have little to no training in, or exposure to treatments other than drugs or surgery.

They aren't trained in preventing disease...

Another example of medical facts reversed is the diet industry. First, a low-calorie diet was said to be the only way to lose weight. Then experts said, "It's not the calories, but the amount of fat you consume that will determine your weight." Now the rage of the day is "It's not the calories and it's not the fat, it's sugar and the high-glycemic carbohydrates that cause obesity." The fact is, nobody really knows.

A hundred years ago people believed they knew all there was about the cure and prevention of disease. We look back at them and we're amazed at just how little they really knew. We laugh at the thought of something like bloodletting curing a disease. Well, guess what? Fifty years from now people will laugh when they look at some of the archaic and horrible so-called cures that we're using today.

I realize that as more research and data become available, there's an excellent chance that many of the theories and opinions I've included in this book may be modified, improved, or even changed completely. Well, since there are virtually no medical facts, only medical opinions, you'll need to choose the opinion that makes the best sense for you.

How did I come up with my opinions? I've traveled over five million miles to bring you this information. I've been in all fifty states in the U.S. and traveled to countries all over the world. Over the last twenty years I have talked with thousands of healthcare providers. I've listened to tens of thousands of people who've had serious medical conditions cured by natural therapies; many after drugs and surgery had failed them.

I have so much firsthand experience with this that I believe I have the unique perspective necessary to come up with my bold conclusions. The biggest acknowledgment I must give is to the tens of thousands of dedicated healthcare professionals around the world who refuse to use drugs and surgery, yet routinely see their patients cured of diseases and go on to live vibrant healthy lives. These natural healthcare providers see people cured of cancer, diabetes, heart disease, chronic pain, headaches, arthritis, allergies, depression, and the list goes on.

The question is no longer whether diseases can be prevented or cured faster and more effectively without drugs and surgery. The real question is why are healthcare providers, who do not use drugs and surgery, being prosecuted as criminals because they cure people of cancer, AIDS, and hundreds of other chronic diseases? Natural therapies work. Natural therapies can work better than drugs or surgery. Those who are using natural therapies to cure and prevent disease, and have a higher success rate and fewer adverse side effects than drug or surgical treatments, are being prosecuted for breaking the law. The question is, why are inexpensive, all natural, safe, effective treatments being suppressed? Let's find out…

CHAPTER 2

What's Wrong With Healthcare In America?

Standard medical science is failing. More people are getting medical treatment, taking more drugs, having more diagnostic testing, and having more surgeries than ever before in history. Yet more people are getting sick than ever before. Today you have a higher chance of getting cancer than ever before in history, and yet with many types of cancer you would have the same chance of dying as you did in 1950. I would call that a miserable failure.

The average American has over thirty different prescription and nonprescription drugs in their medicine cabinet. Do you think they're healthy? Obviously not. Who are the real winners in the cure and prevention of disease? It's certainly not those people taking multiple prescriptions every day. The winners are the drug companies and the healthcare companies. The drug companies' profits are at an all-time high.

And let's look at the diet industry:

✔ More people are on diets than ever before.
✔ More people take more diet products than ever before.
✔ More people exercise than ever before.

And yet, according to the Centers for Disease Control and Prevention, more than one-third (35.7%) of adults living in America are obese. Not just a bit overweight, but obese.

Who are the winners in the war on obesity? The corporations that sell diet food, diet pills, and other weight loss aids, that's who!

What should (and could) the state of our health and fitness look like? An ideal scenario would be one where you never have to take a single drug and you never get sick. You wake up in the morning feeling great, full of energy and vitality. You go throughout your day with a bounce in your step and a smile on your face. You don't feel stressed, anxious, or depressed. You don't feel tired. You've got no headaches or pain in your body. You aren't overweight, and you don't get colds, or the flu, or other illnesses.

> We're also brainwashed into believing that it's "natural" to take drugs.

You're not ravenous with your appetite. You eat what you want and you're never that hungry. You don't deprive yourself of the foods you enjoy. You go to sleep and get a wonderful full night's rest. Your sexual desires are healthy and strong, and you're capable of both giving and receiving sexual pleasure. Your skin, hair, and nails look healthy and radiant. You have strength and tone in your muscles. Your body is graceful and flexible. You're firm, strong, vibrant, and you feel great! That's the description of a healthy person.

Most people have no idea how good their body is designed to feel. We've been brainwashed into believing that it's natural for a human being to get colds and flu, have aches and pains, and other medical problems. You do not have to get sick. Being sick is not "normal," it's abnormal. We're also brainwashed into believing that it's "natural" to take drugs. We're programmed to believe that we "need" drugs in order to be healthy.

Is there a place for surgery and drugs? Sure. Medical science has done a very good job at addressing symptoms. However, the treatment of a symptom has two flaws. First, the treatment itself often causes more problems, which then have to be treated. Second, the cause of the symptom is usually never addressed. When you don't address the cause, you're setting up more problems later on. That said, if you're in an emergency situation like a bad accident, of course drugs and surgery can save your life. However, drugs and surgery have failed at preventing illness and they do not address the cause of illness. If you fall off a ladder and puncture a kidney, of course you want to be rushed to the nearest emergency room and have a trained doctor use drugs and surgery to save your life. But if you want to stay healthy and never have disease, drugs and surgery are not the answer.

So, if trillions of dollars in scientific research has failed to produce ways of preventing and curing illness and disease, and all natural inexpensive prevention methods and cures exist, why aren't we hearing about them? The answer may surprise you.

CHAPTER 3

It's All About the Money

My contention is that there are all natural cures for virtually every ailment. These cures are being hidden from you by the pharmaceutical industry, the Food and Drug Administration, and the Federal Trade Commission, as well as other groups. The question that arises most often when I make this statement is, "Why? What is the motive for such a thing to occur?" The answer is simple: money and power.

All publicly traded corporations have a legal responsibility to increase profits. It's the law. Think about it: The only way companies make increased profits is by producing their product at the lowest possible cost, selling it at the highest possible price, and selling as much as they possibly can. Every decision a company makes is to increase profits.

In business, is everything always about the money? Yes. Throughout the history of big business, planned obsolescence has been standard operating procedure. This is when a product is manufactured in such a way that it will wear out or need to be replaced. The product could have been made to last a long time;

but in order for the company to ensure future profits, it knowingly manufactured an item that was inherently flawed. Thus it planned for the product's obsolescence, all in the name of profit.

Consider the drug industry. Let's say you sell insulin to diabetics. Would you be happy if someone discovered an herb that cured a person's diabetes so that they never needed insulin again? Of course not. You'd be out of business. Healthcare, defined as the treatment, prevention, and diagnosis of disease, is the most profitable industry in the world. As long as people are sick, billions of dollars in profit are made every year. There are enormous amounts of money to be made as long as people stay sick. A healthy person, on the other hand, does not need to buy drugs, doesn't get medical treatment, and is therefore a liability to the corporations involved in healthcare. If every person were healthy and disease-free, the drug companies and virtually the entire healthcare industry would be out of business.

> This money machine does not make its profits by keeping people healthy...

To the drug companies and the corporations involved in healthcare, as long as you're sick, there's money to be made; you're a potentially good customer. There's no financial incentive for the healthcare industry to prevent or cure disease, because the industry is driven to make money.

Let's examine a fictitious (or maybe not so fictitious) scenario. Imagine there's a scientist working in a lab somewhere who makes a breakthrough discovery: a small plant is found in the Amazon that, when brewed into a tea and consumed, eliminates all cancer in the body within one week.

Imagine this researcher proclaiming that he has given this tea to one thousand cancer patients and that every single one of them, within a week and without having undergone surgery, was found to have absolutely no cancer in their body. Eureka! A cure for cancer! An inexpensive, simple plant that you make into a tea and drink. It's all natural, has no side effects, and costs pennies.

Imagine this scientist announcing his discovery to the world. Certainly he'd win a Nobel Prize, right? Certainly the world medical community would be rejoicing. No more cancer!

Unfortunately, you'll never hear this story. Not because it isn't true, but because if a simple herbal tea that cured all cancer was being sold there would be no need for the American Cancer Society. No need for any of the drug companies that manufacture and sell cancer drugs. There would be no need for any cancer research funding. Cancer clinics around the world would close. Hundreds of thousands of people would be put out of work. Entire industries would shut down and billions of dollars in profit would no longer be funneling in to the kingpins who control the cancer industry.

So if such a person made this discovery, what do you think would happen? In some cases these people simply vanish. In others, they're given hundreds of millions of dollars for their research. And in still other cases the federal government raids these researchers' offices, confiscates the data, and jails them for practicing medicine without a license. Is this fantasy or is it the truth? Well, the healthcare industry has a dirty little secret, and I am blowing the whistle on it.

It's all about the money. Hospitals, drug companies, and the entire healthcare industry should really be called the "sick care" industry. This money machine does not make its profits by keeping people healthy, but rather by finding sick people and then selling them their outrageously expensive drugs and medical procedures. And they make over $1.3 trillion annually doing it. I've listened to these people. I've heard CEOs of major pharmaceutical companies say things like, "I don't care how much liver damage this drug causes, get it approved by the FDA. Do it and our stock price goes up threefold."

That is why I am mad as hell, and I am not going to take it anymore. Is it always just about the money? Are natural remedies and cures being suppressed and hidden just because greedy people and corporations want to make more money? Is it true that money makes the world go 'round? Yes. You must understand that the number one motivator in the world is making money. So let's look at who's involved…

CHAPTER 4

Who Are They?

Drugs and surgery are being promoted as the only answer to the prevention and cure of illness and disease. Natural cures are being suppressed and hidden from the public. So who's involved in this cover up?

✔ **The Pharmaceutical Companies.** These include not only the companies that sell drugs, but also companies that research and develop drugs. It also includes the suppliers in the healthcare industry who provide things like syringes, gauze, medical tape, tubing, plastic bottles, tongue depressors, etc. The profits this group of companies makes is astronomical.

✔ **The Food Companies**. You may ask: how do food companies get involved in healthcare? Well, there's a huge correlation between food and healthcare. Keep in mind many food companies are directly or indirectly involved in the pharmaceutical industry through corporate ownership, affiliated business transactions, or by the officers and directors owning stock in the pharmaceutical companies. Food companies include those that manufacture and sell food, and they also include fast food restaurants and the suppliers of the food industry—the actual growers of the food.

✔ **The Trade Associations.** The number of associations involved in the healthcare industry is enormous. Keep in mind, these associations are not in place to eliminate disease or keep people healthy. When you read their charters you find that they are there to promote the disease in an effort to get additional funding, and to protect their members, which are the drug companies and doctors! You've heard of some of them: American Medical Association, American Heart Association, American Lung Association, or American Cancer Society. There are many more than you probably know of—countless numbers of them. You might not be aware that these associations are incredibly powerful. Remember, these are not organizations with a goal of curing and preventing disease, or protecting the consumer. These associations don't represent sick people, they represent their members: The companies, the corporations, and the people making the money. And the people running these associations, of course, have an interest in keeping their cushy jobs.

✔ **Charities and Foundations.** These organizations sound great, but have you met the people who run them? The officers and directors of most charities and foundations have huge salaries and enormous expense accounts. They usually fly first-class, sometimes on private jets. They stay in the most expensive hotels and eat in the finest restaurants with your donations. Some foundations and charities have been found to spend over 40 percent of all of their donations on "administrative costs." Think about it. If a foundation used the money it received to cure a disease, there'd be no further need for the foundation. Consider this: the Jerry Lewis Telethon has raised over $1 billion for muscular dystrophy, yet more people have muscular dystrophy today than ever before.

✔ **Lobbyists**. This is the hidden, secret group of people in Washington that most of you have no idea even exists. These people make on average between $300,000 to $400,000 a year, plus hundreds of thousands more in perks. Their job is simply to walk up to a congressman or senator and try to persuade them to pass a certain piece of legislation, or vote a certain way. How do they do that? Well, the lobbyist can't walk up to a member of Congress and say, "Please vote a certain way on this bill and I'll give you 200,000 dollars." That would be called a bribe. But what the lobbyist can do is say, "Do you have a son or a daughter, Mr. Congressman? You do? Fantastic. I know your son or daughter has absolutely no experience whatsoever, but we'd like to give your son or daughter a job for $200,000 a year. And the best part is they don't even have to show up for work. Oh, by the way Mr. Congressman, would you please vote a certain way on this particular piece of legislation which helps who I represent?" Lobbyists absolutely bribe members of Congress, although Congress has passed laws that make these bribes legally not bribes, by disguising them as other things. Lobbyists may make huge donations to a congressman's favorite charity or school or hire companies that the congressman is affiliated with. Folks, that's what is happening in Washington. But according to the law it's not called a bribe or payoff, it's technically legal. And who made the law? The congressmen. Hmm, pretty interesting, isn't it? They make a law to make sure that what they do is legal.

✔ **Government Agencies**. Primarily the Food and Drug Administration (FDA) and the Federal Trade Commission (FTC). Isn't it surprising that it's the Food AND Drug Administration? (Why not two separate agencies?) This organization is one of the most powerful organizations in the country. They use Gestapo-like tactics to put natural cures out of business. They act as judge, jury, and executioner. They raid companies, unannounced, to seize products such as herbal remedies, vitamins and minerals, computers, files, research data, and equipment. They conduct these raids with armed agents with guns drawn. They seize harmless products, papers, documents, and computers without provocation, with no customer or consumer complaints, and without warning.

Let's look now at how these organizations make it all about the money.

Legal responsibility to shareholders

Virtually every pharmaceutical company is a publicly traded company, which means that the officers and directors have a legal responsibility to increase shareholder value. That means that the officers and directors of virtually every pharmaceutical company have a legal responsibility to increase profits. The only way they can increase profits is to sell more of what they sell and produce those products at a lower cost. Drug companies, therefore, have one goal: To sell more drugs and produce those drugs as inexpensively as possible. Once a drug is approved and the pharmaceutical company has the patent, it becomes the only company that can sell that drug. Getting a patented drug is an automatic billion dollars in the bank. This is why you will never see a pharmaceutical company promoting a natural cure. Natural cures cannot be patented. You can only make profits if you have a patented drug. There are no large profits in selling a natural cure that can't be patented. When you have a patented product you are the only company that can sell it. There's no competition. But if you're selling a natural product, a hundred other companies could sell the same product! Because of that competition, the prices will come down and the profits are reduced. That is why the drug industry will only promote patented drugs, because that's where the profits are. This is also why the drug companies gave tens of millions of dollars to lobbyists to get the FDA to make a new "law." Listen to this carefully. The FDA has the power to make laws and enforce them. It can make these laws without congressional approval or debate. In order to protect the profits of the drug industry the FDA passed the most incredibly insane law of all time. And here it is: "Only a drug can cure, prevent or treat a disease." Think about the ramifications. The FDA has now guaranteed and protected the profits of the drug companies! Only a patented drug, according to the FDA, can treat, prevent, or cure a disease. First off, we

> The pharmaceutical companies give huge cash incentives and information to the doctors...

know this is blatantly untrue. The disease scurvy, for example, which is simply a vitamin C deficiency, is treated, prevented, and cured by eating citrus fruit. According to the FDA's law, however, if you were to holdup an orange and say, "This orange is the cure for the disease of scurvy," you would go to jail for selling a "drug" without a license. I'm not kidding. According to the FDA, as soon as you made a disease claim in reference to taking an orange, the orange was no longer an orange, but magically became a "drug" according to the FDA. And since that "drug" has not been patented or approved by the FDA, you are selling a "drug" without a license, which is a criminal offense. This is how the FDA works to protect the profits of the pharmaceutical company and suppress and hide information about natural remedies.

And just when you think it being all about the money can't get any worse, it does.

Manipulation

You are being duped into buying their drugs. Let's look at how the drug companies accomplish this. Years ago, they basically had to make sure that you were sick and had a problem that a drug could ameliorate. Second, they had to make sure that the doctors prescribed their particular drug. That still goes on. The pharmaceutical companies give huge cash incentives and information to the doctors about the drugs they make to ensure that the doctors, who are in fact legal drug pushers, get their drugs to you via prescription. Remember, the pharmaceutical companies have ensured that you're sick. How do they do that? This is going to blow your mind, but it's sadly true. One of the major reasons there's so much sickness and disease is because of the poisons you are putting in your body. The number one poison you put in your body consists of prescription and nonprescription drugs! That's right. The prescription and nonprescription drugs you're taking to eliminate your symptoms are, in fact, one of the major reasons that you get sick. The pharmaceutical companies know that all drugs have side effects. This is the dirty little secret they don't want you to know. Just as the tobacco industry knew that cigarettes were addictive and could cause lung cancer, yet lied for decades about this fact, the pharmaceutical industry today knows that all drugs have negative side effects and can cause further illness.

Why is the drug industry keeping this information secret? Because it's profitable. Look at the cycle: You start taking a drug to handle a certain symptom. A few months later you develop another medical condition. This new condition, unknown to you, was actually caused by the first drug you were taking. You start taking another drug for this new medical condition. The drug seems to work. Your condition gets better. A few months later, you develop yet another series of medical problems. And you're given still more drugs for the latest conditions… See how profitable this is? The cycle guarantees additional drug sales and profits for the drug companies.

Do you wonder how this is allowed to go on? I'll tell you: Virtually all drug research is funded by the pharmaceutical industry itself, that's how. And in nearly every study, drugs are found to be safe and effective. But of course, that's not true. Think of all of the drugs that were once proven to be safe and effective and approved by the FDA. Then, years later, these same drugs were found to be dangerous. They caused all kinds of severe medical conditions, which then led the FDA to take them off the market. Interestingly enough, they were only taken off the market after the drug companies made millions of dollars in profits.

Advertising

Another way you're being manipulated by it being all about the money is that the pharmaceutical industry is doing something that it hadn't done historically—advertising its drugs directly to the consumer. Close to two-thirds of all advertising in America is for drugs. It's estimated that the drug industry spends well in excess of $10 billion a year on advertising. These ads show beautiful, happy people, and give you the impression that they're taking this wonderful drug and that their lives are so much better. They're actors. Even when well-known figures and famous actors publicly endorse a drug or foundation (usually funded by pharmaceutical companies), ostensibly because they or a close friend or relative has suffered with a particular disease, they're being paid enormous sums to do so. These ads are not truthful.

Collusion

The Food and Drug Administration, the Federal Trade Commission and the pharmaceutical industry have an unholy alliance. The regulating government body should be governing, regulating and protecting consumers from the drug companies' insatiable desire to make profits. But it isn't. They work together to increase profits and power. A law was passed in Congress with virtually no debate which increased the FDA's dependence on large drug companies for its funding. Yes, you read that correctly. The FDA gets funding directly from the drug industry. And guess who owns stock in these drug companies? Would it surprise you that many members of the FDA and FTC own stock in drug companies? Would it surprise you that many members of Congress own stock in drug companies? Would it also surprise you that members of the news media, that are supposed to be impartially presenting news, own stock in drug companies? And the corporations that own television networks, radio networks, newspapers, and magazines all have financial ties to the pharmaceutical industry? That's one of the reasons you hear so much about drugs on the news and read so many positive articles about them in magazines and newspapers. These organizations get financial benefit from the drugs they help to sell.

> The FDA gets funding directly from the drug industry.

Doesn't it surprise you that you almost never hear any positive news about an herbal remedy, a natural remedy, or a homeopathic remedy in mainstream media? Could it be that there's no profit in those remedies? Remember, natural remedies cannot be patented.

The FDA says that there is not, and never will be, a natural remedy that can cure, prevent, or treat a disease. Because if a natural remedy did, then it would have to be classified as a "drug" and once it's classified as a drug it has to go through 800 million dollars' worth of testing that the FDA requires to approve it as a new drug. This cannot be done. Why? Because a natural remedy cannot be patented and there's no company that can spend $800 million to get a natural remedy approved as a new drug because it won't own a patent for that drug and therefore can't make that money back plus tenfold profits. This is why the FDA and drug companies love this system. It prevents any natural remedy from being touted as a cure or preventative of disease when in fact many of them are.

Can you see how the pharmaceutical industry is committed to wiping out non-patentable, all natural cures for disease? It's spending hundreds of millions of dollars to try to get you to believe that drugs are safe and effective and all natural cures are ineffective and dangerous. It's the drugs that are dangerous and cause disease. And the current research shows that drugs do not cure disease either. Natural remedies are generally safe, effective, and have virtually no side effects. Technically, all natural remedies do not cure disease either, because only the body can do that. But these remedies help the body cure itself.

Government Mandates of Drug Use

Another technique that the drug industry uses to make sure sales of drugs continue to increase is to get the federal government to pass laws requiring people to take drugs. There are three methods employed. First, pass a law requiring that children must take a certain drug, such as vaccines. Second, pass a law requiring all federal employees and military personnel to take a certain drug. Third, get the government to pay for drug usage for the poor and elderly through Social Security, Medicare, and Medicaid. When this happens…bam! Billions of dollars in profits.

Censorship of Opposing Ideas

We live in America—the supposed land of free speech. Well, speech is not free. If your speech happens to threaten the profits of big business, you are going to be bound, gagged, ridiculed and persecuted. A plethora of books is written about the drug industry, the FDA, the FTC, and the collusion between the associations, corporations, lobbyists, and certain government regulators and how they work together to suppress natural, inexpensive ways to prevent and cure disease. But they rarely, if ever, get published, because if a publisher puts out a book that's bashing the pharmaceutical industry, or certain government agencies, or big business, the publishing company may be blacklisted and have its other books taken out of distribution, which would cost them millions of dollars in profits.

And it's not just books that are censored. News organizations will block unflattering stories involving these companies, too. Several years ago, a couple of reporters did an exposé on the company now infamous for genetically modifying (and ruining) our food: Monsanto. This story was about the growth hormone rBGH that's used in dairy cows. It revealed that this hormone was making the animals sick and making the milk and dairy products from these cows poisonous. However, the news organization they wrote the story for refused to run it and tried to pay them hush money. Why? Because Monsanto put pressure on the news organization!

Censorship of Advertising

Let's say you're the president of a major television network. The network is owned by another multinational company that owns a drug company, or has a huge interest in one. Your network gets two-thirds, or close to 70 percent, of its advertising revenue directly from the drug industry. Now imagine a guy comes to you and says, "I'd like to advertise my book entitled *How the Drug Companies Are Ripping Off America*." Would you, as the president of that company, run that ad? Of course not. You'd get fired. Because that ad could have a negative impact on the sales and profits of the drug companies in which the owner of the network has a major equity position. Folks, this is what is happening. *It's all about the money.*

Debunking Natural Remedies

In an actual memorandum, the U.S. federal government states that one of the most effective tools to get people to believe the government's opinion is to put together a well-orchestrated debunking campaign. What this means is there is a coordinated effort between the FDA, the FTC, the healthcare associations, and the entire pharmaceutical industry as well as some major news organizations to produce scare tactic stories about natural alternatives and suppress the truth about the ineffectiveness and dangers of drugs. There's a litany of inexpensive, highly effective natural cures that are being labeled as "snake oil" or simply hidden from the public.

The FDA has led the way in this battle against natural cures. In the 1970s the FDA attempted to make vitamin supplements prescription drugs. They claimed that vitamins were so dangerous they should only be prescribed by doctors. The public was outraged and Congress rejected the idea. In 1993 the FDA tried to classify certain minerals and amino acids as prescription drugs. Again, a public outcry caused Congress to act. The FDA has gone after companies that sell natural remedies via the Internet. It claims these companies are selling "drugs" without a license.

In 2013 an *Associated Press* story claimed that vitamins and food supplements were deemed ineffective. Here's a quote from this story: "The government doesn't recommend routine vitamin supplementation as a way to prevent chronic diseases."

The article later quotes a medical doctor who says, "Most people who buy multivitamins and other supplements are generally healthy." Exactly. So, the doctor, along with the government, recommends that they stop? Sounds ludicrous, but I am not making this up.

There are thousands of studies showing that natural remedies are not only effective, but they can be more effective than a drug counterpart. An example is Vitamin E. In major double-blind studies, Vitamin E was found as effective or more effective as a blood thinner than its drug counterpart. But why aren't we given Vitamin E instead of the drug? The facts are clear: natural remedies could financially devastate the pharmaceutical industry.

Did you know that there are different standards used in what's classified as news and advertising? If information is presented by a politician or government agency, such as the FDA or FTC, news organizations present that information as factual, rarely if ever investigating the claims or seeking an opposing viewpoint. The government has the ability to influence the masses without opposition.

Lawsuits

The industry uses lawsuits to spread negative information about natural remedies. Keep in mind the pharmaceutical industry is the most powerful, profitable business in the world. It can afford to file outrageous, frivolous lawsuits against small independent companies that threaten profits, and drive them right out of business.

Lawsuits are also routinely filed against individual healthcare practitioners who are curing people without drugs or surgery. Not only are civil lawsuits filed against them, but many of these health-care providers are being prosecuted criminally for curing people's diseases. They're being charged with practicing medicine without a license or dispensing drugs without a license.

The bottom line is that there are natural, inexpensive, safe cures for almost every disease. The pharmaceutical industry, the FTC, the FDA and the rest of "them" are suppressing this information. The pharmaceutical industry, the drug industry, the food industry, the associations and government agencies, all have a major financial incentive to keep people sick. There are billions of dollars in profits as long as people stay sick and there are billions of dollars in profits as long as people take more and more drugs. Remember, it's always all about the money!

So if we can't believe our government; if we can't believe what we see on television, or what we hear on the radio, or what we read in newspapers and magazines; if we can't believe what we hear from professors and doctors since they're all paid spokespeople for the pharmaceutical industry, then who *can* we believe when it comes to information about health and the treatment, prevention, and cure of disease? It only makes sense that you can't believe anyone who has a financial interest in selling you something. You can't even believe alternative healthcare practitioners who are trying to sell you vitamins. If a licensed healthcare practitioner tells you the benefits of a vitamin, herb, or mineral and he's encouraging you to buy from him at a profit, maybe he's being sincere and truthful, but the financial incentive may impede your ability to get unbiased information. The officers and directors of vitamin, mineral, herb, and homeopathic companies have financial motivations to sell their products just like the officers and directors of pharmaceutical companies. And as long as someone is selling something, it's all about the money. Always.

> And as long as someone is selling something, it's all about the money.

So again, the question is who can you listen to? The answer: You can listen to ME! You might laugh, but it's true.

People all around the world come up to me and ask, "Where do I go for information about health? Who can I trust? Where can I get information about the prevention or curing of a disease? There's so much conflicting information out there, and I just don't know where to go to find the answers." This is the big problem. With the Internet there is more information available than ever before, but when you go on online everyone is trying to sell you something. So when you're reading an article you don't know if the information is true, or just designed to get you to buy a product. WebMD is a perfect example. This is a publicly traded company where the officers and directors have made millions of dollars in profits.

WebMD, in my opinion, is nothing more than a front for the pharmaceutical industry encouraging you to buy and use drugs and get expensive medical procedures. It tries to make you think it's an unbiased source of information when this is categorically untrue. How can they be unbiased when they accept advertising from drug companies? How can they be unbiased when they're publicly traded? How can they be unbiased when their only motivation is to make money?

What makes me different? The answer is simple. For me, it's not all about the money. It's not that I think making money is bad. Giving a good quality service at a good value is an admirable thing to do. Making a profit and enjoying a beautiful lifestyle is not bad. Making money at the expense of employees, customers and the environment is bad.

Here is how I've solved the problem: I do not take any advertising. I do not sell any natural cure products: I only inform. And that's why you can listen to what I am saying in this book, on my website www.NaturalCuresBook.com, and in my newsletter that you can subscribe to by going to www.NaturalCuresBook.com/newsletter.

People approach me regularly offering me money to endorse their product, to recommend their product, or to talk positively about one product, or bash another, but I'm not interested in that. What I'm interested in is sharing information that helps people. So let's get on with that....

CHAPTER 5

Why Are We Sick?

Over the years, the pharmaceutical industry has come up with different theories about why people get sick. Antibiotics were touted as the cure all. The theory was that all disease was caused by germs, primarily bacteria. This theory has been proven wrong. Stronger and stronger antibiotics continue to be developed, and yet people continue to get sicker, and sicker. More people are getting more diseases than ever before.

The next theory was that viruses were the cause of all illness and disease. Unfortunately, few people know that antibiotics have no effect on viruses. The doctors continually prescribe antibiotics at the drop of a hat. People have been brainwashed into thinking they need antibiotics when they feel sick, so they demand them. Doctors, who are in business to make money, understand that patients are essentially customers and so to keep the customers happy they prescribe the antibiotics. According to the Associated Press it's estimated that about half of the antibiotic prescriptions written each year are unnecessary. Still, people continue to get more sicknesses and diseases.

One current theory is that a large percentage of disease and illness is caused by genetic defects. Of course they tell us the only answer is drugs. A new method of making billions of dollars is to come up with a genetic defect for every problem a person has. "Oh, you're fat because you have a genetic defect, and a drug is being worked on that can solve that genetic defect and make you thin." "Diabetes is nothing more than genetics, so we'll work on a drug that will correct that genetic disposition." Keep in mind that drug companies really do *not* want to cure disease as they claim. If they came up with a cure, they'd be out of business.

> If they came up with a cure, they'd be out of business.

Take herpes for example. Herpes is a virus. Ads on TV regularly say there is no cure for herpes, therefore, in order to suppress the symptoms, take our wonderful drug every day for the rest of your life. Imagine what would happen to the publicly traded company that makes the drug if they announced, "Here is a cure for herpes. Simply take this herb for thirty days and you'll never have a herpetic breakout ever again. By the way, this herb is not patented and it costs only three dollars."

That company would lose billions of dollars in profits. Its stock price would plummet. Therefore, there's no incentive to cure herpes. The incentive is to keep the public brainwashed into believing there is no cure for herpes, and the only solution to the "symptoms" is drugs. Remember, the FDA and the drug companies work hand in hand. If I happen to know a cure for herpes, I can't say so. Because if I *do* I'm now making a medical claim and, according to the FDA, I'm breaking the law. Even if what I'm saying is true, I am still breaking the law. The FDA will then come in with their federal agents with their guns drawn, arrest me, throw me in jail, confiscate any papers I have, and any of the harmless herb, suppress the information and outlaw it because there is no "credible scientific evidence." They will then put out press releases stating that

I'm a charlatan selling snake oil and have no scientific evidence to substantiate my claim. Unfortunately, that's how the system works.

So why do you get sick? Is it germs? Bacteria? Is it viruses? Genetics? Well let's think about it. You don't *catch* cancer. Your body develops cancer. You don't catch diabetes. Your body develops diabetes. You don't catch obesity. Your body becomes obese. You don't catch headaches, fibromyalgia, arthritis, PMS, or impotence. These are conditions that develop within the body. They're not caused by a germ, or a virus. Drugs are not the answer. You don't have a headache because you have an aspirin deficiency. The question is why do human beings have so much illness? Is there a way that we can do some simple things to keep us illness free, and full of life, energy, and vitality? Yes.

Let's go back to the cause of all disease and the reason why we're sick. Based on personal experience, reading thousands of pages of documents, and hearing the firsthand accounts from thousands of people and healthcare practitioners around the world, I've come up with what I believe to be the cause of virtually all sickness and disease in the body. There are two main reasons why you get sick:

1. You "catch" something. This means your body picked up a "germ," generally a virus or bacteria.

2. You "develop" an illness or disease. This means there is some imbalance in the body, something is not working right.

Common diseases in this category include: cancer, diabetes, acid reflux, arthritis, heart disease, etc. In our search for the ultimate cause of all illness and the ultimate cure for all illnesses, we need to ask, "What caused that?" With this in mind, let's start with "catching something."

One may say that the "cause" of catching a germ is pretty evident. You obviously caught the germ from someone else who had it. This is where medical science stops. They claim that drugs must be developed in order to kill those bacteria and viruses. However, they're asking the wrong question. The fact is that we're *all* exposed to bacteria and viruses *daily*. If one person in your home or office has the flu, then every single person has been exposed to the flu virus. Some people succumb to bacteria and viruses and get sick, and others don't. Throughout your life you'll pick up thousands of bacteria and viruses. That's natural. Why, in some cases, does the body not do what it was designed to do, which is fight off the bacteria or virus? The answer: the body is out of balance and the immune system is weak.

When your body is in balance (a state called homeostasis), and your immune system is strong, you don't develop any symptoms of the viruses or bacteria that you pick up.

Now the question becomes, "What is causing the body to be out of balance, and the immune system to be weak?" I'll give you the answer in a moment, but first let's go to the second reason people get sick. Remember, you get sick because you either a) catch something, or b) something develops in the body.

You "catch something" because your body is out of balance and your immune system is weak. You "develop something" either because your body is out of balance, or a "toxin" is getting into your body causing the problem to develop.

If we keep asking the question, "What caused that..." we can then conclude that all your illness comes from one of, or a combination of the following things:

1. You have too many toxins in your body.

2. You have nutritional deficiencies.

3. You are exposed to, and negatively affected by electromagnetic chaos.

4. You have trapped mental and emotional stress.

These are the only four reasons why your immune system could be weak or why genetically weak areas in the body can break down, thus allowing illness and disease to develop. These four things cause the body to be "out of balance." I will address each of these four issues.

Let's start with toxins. What is a toxin? A toxin is a poison. It is a substance that if taken in large doses can cause severe illness or death. In relation to toxins, the question is what is causing toxins to be put into our body? The answer is that we have not been educated to know what these toxins are. And secondly, these toxins are being put in virtually everything we eat without our knowledge.

Now, here is the big one: the most toxic thing you can put in your body, and the number one cause of virtually all illness and disease, is prescription and nonprescription drugs!

In my opinion, one of the main reasons people are sick is because of the number of drugs they take. Why? Because *all* drugs have negative side effects. Let me say it again, all drugs have negative side effects! If you're taking a drug to suppress one symptom, that drug is causing some other problem to start developing in your body.

Even if you stop taking that drug, the wheels have been set in motion, and in a few weeks, or a few months, boom, you have some more symptoms caused by the first drug you took a few months ago. You go to your doctor, and he or she gives you another drug to suppress these new symptoms. This *new* drug has negative side effects, and after you start taking it, again, the wheels will have been set in motion, and *voila*—new symptoms which were in fact caused by the drug you were just taking. You go back to the doctor and get another drug...

Drugs...Cause...Medical...Problems. They do not treat the cause. It's a great business for the drug companies, not so great for you. If they get you taking one drug, they've got you. The likelihood of you taking another drug, and then another, keeps going up and up. The more you take, the sicker you get, simply because drugs are major toxins.

I know some of you are saying, "Drugs can't really be poison, can they?" Oh no? Then how about you take thirty of them right now and see what happens? You'll probably die. If you eat thirty apples are you going to die? Not likely. You may feel full, and you might need to go to the bathroom a lot, but you're probably going to survive an apple overdose.

This relates to nonprescription over-the-counter drugs as well. Let me be very clear. The scary thing is the drug companies and the FDA know it.

A good example of this is Vioxx. Vioxx is a pain medication. It was an outrageously expensive drug that reduced pain no better than an over-the-counter drug. The drug company that sold Vioxx made billions in profits. Whistleblowers now say that both the FDA and the drug manufacturer of Vioxx knew it would cause over 100,000 people to die. Whistleblowers say that the decision was made to let the people die because of the potential profits. In my opinion, this happens all of the time. Over-the-counter drugs are some of the biggest culprits. Many of these drugs were approved by the FDA twenty, thirty, forty years ago. The problem is once a drug is approved by the FDA, whether it's a prescription drug or a nonprescription drug, there is virtually no follow-up research or testing to verify the long-term effectiveness of the drug and the long-term safety. We're seeing now that over-the-counter drugs that have been sold for thirty years are being looked at by some independent organizations and they're being shown to be dangerous and ineffective. They're also being shown to cause illness and disease.

Cholesterol lowering drugs, for example, have an adverse effect on the liver. The liver is the only fat metabolizing organ in the body. The liver is needed for proper body function. When the liver is adversely affected you are prone to diabetes, acid reflux, constipation, colon cancer, heart disease, asthma, arthritis, and dozens of other illnesses and disease.

Do cholesterol-lowering drugs directly cause these illnesses and disease? No one really knows for sure, but it's certainly obvious to anyone with half a brain and a little bit of logic that these absolutely contribute to the development of disease in the body.

> All drugs have negative side effects.

The bottom line is all over-the-counter nonprescription drugs and prescription drugs cause illness and disease. This is the big shocker. The industry that's promoting itself as the group dedicated to the prevention and cure of disease is actually the group causing more sickness and disease. All drugs are chemicals. All drugs have negative side effects. All drugs can cause death. All drugs are poisons. Did you know that more Americans die every year from prescription drugs than from illegal drugs? There are dozens of articles showing how prescription and nonprescription drugs are causing all illness and diseases.

Drugs are toxins. When one has lots of toxins in the body, the body goes out of balance. The immune system is weakened. When this occurs the body cannot fight off the viruses or bacteria that it picks up, thus causing sickness.

"Too many toxins in the body" comes down to this:

1. What goes into the body.
2. What comes out of the body.
3. Exercise.

4. Rest.

5. Thoughts.

6. What you say.

Let's go through this list and address some common misconceptions, and see what you should be doing if you want to eliminate disease. Maybe some of you have a disease or know someone who does. Others may be concerned about getting a disease and want to do the steps necessary to prevent one.

The six areas listed above have a direct relation to toxicity in the body. It's interesting to note that when you are toxic, your body becomes highly acidic. Your body pH should be alkaline. When your body pH is acidic you are susceptible to illness and disease. When your body pH is alkaline, you virtually never get sick. Every single person who has cancer has a pH that is too acidic.

Let me show you how each of the above six areas cause you to become too toxic, thus more acidic, and thus more prone to illness and disease.

What Goes Into the Body

Let's look at what we put into our bodies. We put things into the body in a variety of ways, but mostly through the mouth. Jack LaLane, who was vibrant, healthy and strong well into his nineties before he passed away at ninety-six said it best: "If man made it, don't eat it." What you put into your mouth should be as close as possible to what nature intended. If you go out and eat an apple you may think, "Ah, this is an apple; man didn't make it, so I can eat it." Well, unfortunately there's a problem with that, because many fruits and vegetables today are man-made.

I mentioned Monsanto in an earlier chapter. You've probably heard news in the past couple of years about this huge chemical and agricultural biotechnology company and its genetically modified food. Some say Monsanto is the devil incarnate and I can't say that I disagree. Monsanto supplies a lot of our nation's food, and much of it, including fruits and vegetables, have been genetically modified to become more disease resistant. Remember what I said about the pharmaceutical industry being all about the money? Well, the food industry is all about the money, too.

A food manufacturer, or for that matter a farmer, is in business and has to sell more of his product and produce at the lowest possible cost to make more money. So farmers say, "Hmm, how can I grow the largest yield of apples or carrots, or the most onions on my field? How can I produce them in the shortest period of time, at the lowest cost, so I can sell them at the highest possible profit?"

The answer is mess around with mother nature and change these natural fruits and vegetables with some man-made concoction that came out of a laboratory so that they grow bigger, faster and more resistant to disease. So through genetic modification, your all natural carrot is no longer all natural. It is really a man-made product.

And it gets worse. Because that farmer has to produce more carrots per acre in order to make more profit, he uses chemical fertilizers and pesticides and herbicides. When you eat that "natural" vegetable or piece of fruit, it's loaded with toxic chemicals. It also has less nutritional value than it would have had fifty or sixty years ago.

So, if you're going to eat fruits and vegetables, which I highly encourage you to do, they must be *organically grown.*

Grains such as rice and oats are the same. Buy organic. I don't recommend wheat or wheat flour *at all*, because wheat in this country has been modified so drastically it's not even the same grain it once was. It's "Frankenwheat," full of "man-made" garbage that will make you sick and fat.

In the United States, nearly all of our fruits, vegetables, grains, nuts and seeds are grown with highly poisonous chemical fertilizers, pesticides and herbicides.

The same conditions apply in the meat industry. Like farmers and other food producers, the meat industry needs to create a lot of product cheaply and quickly in order to sell it for as high a profit as possible. To that end, the industry uses hormones to speed an animal's growth (contributing to the record levels of obesity and early puberty in our children), antibiotics to keep an animal healthy in unsanitary and inhumane conditions, and feeds that are unnatural to an animal's diet that not only pump more chemicals into the meat, but also upset animals' systems so that they become out of balance and diseased, and pass those imbalances and diseases along to those who consume the meat. Remember, if it's not organic, *don't eat it.*

> When you eat that "natural" vegetable or piece of fruit, it's loaded with toxic chemicals.

The same holds true with dairy products. Because of the use of drugs, growth hormones, pasteurization and homogenization, dairy products today are a major health concern unless they're organic, not pasteurized, and not homogenized. Pasteurization simply heats the dairy product to a temperature high enough to kill bacteria. The problem is it also kills the living enzymes, making it harder for our bodies to digest. But more importantly, and more dangerous, is homogenization.

Remember the milkman? You may be too young to remember, but milkmen used to deliver bottled milk to our houses. Why couldn't we just buy our milk in the store? Because back then milk spoiled within just a few days. The food industry said, "We're losing money by not selling milk in our stores. It goes bad too quickly." So they came up with a solution—a process called homogenization. When milk was delivered back in the day the cream separated into a layer on top and you had to shake the bottle to blend it. The process of homogenization actually spins the milk at a high rate breaking down the clusters of molecules within it. As a result, not only does the cream not separate, the milk won't spoil quickly. It can last a couple of weeks before going bad.

The problem with homogenized and pasteurized milk, and other dairy products is that with the processing, the clusters of fat molecules are now so small that when we ingest them they get into our blood stream, which they shouldn't, and our bodies set up a defense mechanism that ends up scarring our arteries. The scarring of the arteries causes LDL cholesterol to attach itself to the artery, which leads to a major cause of heart disease, arteriosclerosis. The processed milk's tiny fat molecules are also being assimilated into the lining of the stomach in a way that's incompatible with our bodies. This clogs the system, making it harder to digest food, which in turn contributes to acid reflux, obesity, allergies, and constipation. The bottom line is pasteurized and homogenized dairy products are unnatural.

When you eat fish you're only slightly better off, because many kinds of fish are "farmed," meaning that toxic feed and chemicals are used to make it grow unnaturally fast and to unnaturally large sizes. When you consume this "man-made" fish, you're also taking in the toxins that have been used in its production. Fish in the wild are ostensibly better. However, because of the massive dumping of poisonous chemicals into our lakes, rivers, and oceans, many wild fish have abnormally high levels of toxic chemicals in them as well.

I know this sounds terrible. I know you're probably wondering *what do I do? How do I eat?* The good news is there are some simple, easy solutions, which I'll explain in a later chapter. I'm trying to point out that you are constantly loading your body with toxins, and this is one of the reasons you get sick. When I tell people they're toxic, most have a hard time believing it, but the fact is you're likely to be toxic right now, just by virtue of the environment.

In 2005, an independent study on women's breast milk showed a startling fact. Virtually all of the women tested, across several states, showed detectable levels of rocket fuel in their breast milk. Yes rocket fuel in breast milk. It wasn't until nearly a decade later in 2013 that NASA announced that it's planning to replace the toxic fuel with a more environmentally friendly one.

We're exposed to environmental toxins constantly. For example when a plane flies overhead there's a "chem-trail." The chemical residues fall down from the sky and we breathe them in. They also contaminate water supplies, which we drink.

What other toxins do we put in our bodies through our mouths? If it's in a box, a jar or a can, it's been processed by the food industry. The food industry puts tens of thousands of chemical ingredients into the food and, in many cases they do not have to list those ingredients on the label. How do they get away with that? They do it through lobbyist friends, and by paying off politicians and members of the Food and Drug Administration. And why is that bad? Because, as I've explained, the additives are toxic. And not only are these chemical additives toxic, when they're put into the food, the processing strips away much of the nutritional value. And in some cases, the additives actually block absorption of nutrients as well.

So, not only are you not getting enough nutrients from the food you're eating, but the few nutrients you are getting are not being absorbed. Why are these food additives put in the food anyway? Well it's very interesting. I was at a health spa where I spoke with a gentleman who was a senior executive at a company that was one of the largest producers of canned goods in the world. We were talking about the food additives and, yes, he admitted that there are thousands and thousands of chemical additives put into the food, and many of these additives are not listed on the label at all. I suggested that these food additives were dangerous to a person's health and were one of the reasons why people are so sick today. He assured me that these chemicals were totally safe, and that they were in such small amounts that they would have no effect on one's body.

I asked, "If they're totally safe, then if I were to give you a glass of one of these chemicals, would you drink it?" He stammered and went back and forth a few times. I must have asked him the question ten times without getting an answer. Finally he said no, he wouldn't drink it because it could potentially be a problem. He admitted that the ingredients were, in fact, toxic. But he repeated that because they were in such small amounts, they had no effect at all on the human body.

I then asked him the million dollar question. I said, "If you're putting such a small amount in, and these ingredients have no effect at all on the human body, then they must have no effect at all on the food. So why do you have to put them in the food?" Again, he couldn't answer. After I continued grilling this man, he reluctantly admitted that they in fact have a major effect. They preserve the food and give it taste. Bingo.

Still, I suspected that there was something else these ingredients did that he wasn't telling. So I searched through my network of insiders, and here is what I discovered: The food industry, just like the tobacco industry, is hiding a dirty little secret. The food industry is putting ingredients in the food purposely, because these secret (and in many cases illegal) ingredients make a person hungry, and make them addicted to the food. Think this is crazy? Remember Coca Cola? Coca Cola was colored sweetened water that had cocaine in it. Coca Cola was the name because Coca referred to the coca plant and Cola referred to the cola nut. The cola nut had the caffeine, and the coca or the cocaine got the person physically addicted. The drug was removed back in the 1920s, without much fanfare or media exposure. Scary, huh? There are more scary things...

Many of the ingredients they put in the food make you depressed, which is good for the drug companies, because if you're depressed, you have to go to the drug companies to treat your depression. Interestingly enough, some of the additives that are put in the food to make you depressed are manufactured by the same companies that sell antidepressant drugs. It's a fantastic business model folks. Remember, it's all about the money.

There's another reason chemical additives and the food processing are bad. Food must have nutritional value for it to be used by the body, but food also has a "vibration." It has a "life force energy." When food is chemically or genetically altered, highly processed, or contains chemical additives, the energetic vibration of the food is altered. When the vibration of food is radically altered consuming that food actually causes the body to go out of balance and causes disease to develop. Yes, you're reading this right. From an energetic standpoint eating a genetically altered apple that's been sprayed with pesticides can give you cancer, as well as dozens of other diseases.

Without giving a physics lesson, when you eat something you're getting the energy from that thing. How do we know this is true? Say you take a pot and you put soil in it. You put in ten pounds of soil, and you put in a little tiny seed, and every day you add some water. Then at the end of a year you have a big plant. Well, take the plant out, shake off the soil from the roots and weigh the soil. Guess what? You still have ten pounds of soil. The only thing you added was some water. If you were to measure the water, you may have added about five pounds of water. Theoretically, the plant should weigh no more than five pounds if it grabbed 100 percent of the water. But the plant weighs fifty pounds. Wow! What happened? How did fifty pounds of mass and matter magically appear? It didn't eat the soil, the ten pounds of soil is still there, and there were only five pounds of water added. How did that plant appear out of virtually nothing? This is a very important point. The plant, like all living things, was created out of "energy." Energy is "invisible matter."

> ...the food industry lobbied the politicians to allow certain man-made ingredients to be classified as all natural.

Human beings are the same. If you take a little baby, and you weigh every bit of food that goes in and then subtract all of the excretions that come out via the urine, stool, and sweat through the skin, you would see that whatever goes in comes out. If ten pounds of food and water are put in, guess what? Ten pounds of stuff comes out. But the baby grows from fifteen pounds to fifty pounds to one hundred and fifty pounds. How does that happen? The answer is that we get the energy from food, from sunlight and from air; and that's how matter is manifested—it's the energy. Everything is energy, including us. We actually become the very energy we take in.

So if we go through everything that we put into our mouth, whatever we eat or drink, we have to ask ourselves is that energy good? Is it as nature intended? Or has it been screwed up by some greedy people who don't care if we get sick?

What should we eat and drink? Ideally you want to eat all natural things, fruits and vegetables, and get them organic. Cooking destroys some of the enzymes, so raw is generally better, but there are some vegetables that are better absorbed when cooked, like tomatoes and carrots. Aim for a hefty amount (between one and two pounds) of organic fruits and vegetables a day. That may sound like a lot, but one piece of fruit can be more than one-fourth a pound. One sweet potato can be one-half a pound.

And don't just look at food labels. You have to read the ingredients. Because even if the label says all natural, that's often a lie. Why? Because the food industry lobbied the politicians to allow certain man-made ingredients to be classified as all natural.

If it's in a box or can, don't even eat it. Buy from the organic section of the grocery store, or better still, buy organic directly from farmer's markets. If you're not eating organic, you're running the risk of ingesting a lot of chemicals that are potentially harmful. These secret chemicals in nonorganic foods are specifically designed to do the following things:

Preserve the food. Sometimes chemicals are added so that food will not spoil even after years of just sitting around. We've all heard the story of the thirty-year-old Twinkie that looked and tasted the same as it did the day it was manufactured.

✔ **Taste and texture.** Much of today's food is produced in such an unnatural way that is has very little nutritional value and very little taste. Chemicals must be added to make the food taste like it's supposed to taste. A major hamburger chain adds a chemical to its hamburgers to make them taste like a hamburger!

✔ **To make you hungry.** The food industry knows that it must sell MORE food to make more money. If it can add a chemical that makes you hungrier, you'll eat more food and they'll make more money!

✔ **To make you fatter.** Fat people eat more food. Chemicals are being added to our food that actually make us gain weight. The more fat people, the more profits for the food industry. Shockingly, one such chemical is actually put into most "diet food." How sad that unknowing consumers buy a product that has the word "diet" on it in the hopes of losing weight, when actually eating it causes them to gain weight.

✔ **To get the person addicted to the product.** Food manufacturers are knowingly putting chemicals into the food that cause the consumer to become physically addicted to it. We know that drugs, which are simply chemicals, can be incredibly physically and emotionally addictive. Having a person addicted to your product is good for profits.

✔ **To give you disease.** As outrageous as it seems, it appears that insiders know that certain "food additives" cause specific diseases. If you knew that huge numbers of people would be coming down with a certain disease in the next five or ten years, you could invest in drug companies that are producing drugs that will be prescribed for this "new disease." When I talk about the greed of the people involved, most people reading this have no comprehension of just how the love of money has taken control over these people's actions, ethics, and morals.

Obviously, what I'm sharing here are my own conclusions. They are vehemently denied by the food industry and the FDA, but think about the same type of denials for years by the tobacco industry. I believe time will prove me correct.

The other important issue relating to these chemical additives is that when you ingest them, they do not necessarily leave your body. Chemical fertilizers, pesticides, herbicides, hormones, prescription and nonprescription drugs, and food additives such as artificial sweeteners, stay in the body and lodge in the fatty tissues. Since our brain is mostly fat, a large percentage of these chemicals accumulate there over the years. This is believed to be one of the main reasons that there's an increase in depression, stress and anxiety, and an increase in learning disabilities like attention deficit disorder. These additives stress the body. When the body is "stressed" two things occur:

1. The immune system is suppressed, making you more susceptible to disease.

2. It can turn your body from the natural alkaline pH state, in which disease and illness and sickness cannot survive, to an acidic state in which diseases like cancer, arteriosclerosis and diabetes can thrive.

When you put something in your mouth ask yourself: Could this have been made a hundred years ago? If it couldn't, don't eat it. The reason it is being processed the way it is, is because somebody is making lots of money. As I've said repeatedly, it's always about the money.

> ...chemical additives...do not necessarily leave your body.

If you were to read the labels of everything you put in your mouth, you would see the names of various chemicals. All of the chemicals listed are dangerous poisons. If you were to ingest a large amount of any of those chemicals at one time, you would probably die.

Now think about the 15,000 chemicals that are in our food that do *not* even have to be listed on the label. Remember, you get sick because you either catch something or you develop something. Catching something is not a problem because your body is designed to fight off infection and disease. But when your body is loaded with toxins (from all those chemicals you're ingesting) and your immune system is suppressed because of lack of nutrition or energetic frequency imbalances, you become susceptible to viruses and bacteria. You develop diseases because toxins, nutritional deficiencies, or energetic imbalances allow disease to form in the genetically weak areas of your system.

It's important to understand why we become ill in order for us to totally understand how to *cure* ourselves. If you really understand why you become sick, then you will understand the "natural cures" much more easily. As I mentioned earlier, this may sound overwhelming. Just go with the flow. The good news is you don't have to be a health fanatic to cure yourself and live a life of health and vitality.

Now let's talk about what else you put in your mouth, primarily what *you drink*. There are two problems here. The first one is most people don't drink enough water, and the second, is that the water you drink is toxic. All tap water has chemicals added to it, primarily chlorine and fluoride, both of which have been found to be toxic.

Most people are dehydrated. Dehydration causes all kinds of medical problems including pain, stiffness, arthritis, asthma, allergies and other medical issues. Dehydration means the cells don't have enough fluid. It can affect your energy and your sleep, but the major thing that it affects is the ability to remove toxins and waste out of the body and out of the cells.

Cells can live forever in a laboratory as long as the fluid in which the cell is living is continually cleaned and changed. If you take a cell and add fluid to it, the cell excretes waste matter and toxins. As long as you clean the environment and get rid of the waste matter and toxins, the cell never seems to age. That's pretty staggering. And it's why removing the toxins from your system is so important. It's also why putting the least amount of toxins *into* your body is so important too.

The debate is on about the best type of water. We have tap water, purified water, spring water and distilled water.

Tap water is absolutely the worst kind, because virtually all tap water is contaminated. All tap water has chlorine in it, and most has synthesized fluoride in it. Synthesized fluoride is toxic.

Most countries in Europe do not have water fluoridation. However, here in the U.S., through lobbying, fluoride was sold to municipalities and dumped in our water supplies under the disguise of being good for our teeth. It isn't true. Even the Centers For Disease Control (CDC) has acknowledged that drinking fluoridated water doesn't benefit teeth. Fluoride is dangerous, and should not be consumed. It adversely affects our organs, primarily the thyroid gland.

Spring water is better than tap water. But certain agencies and interest groups publish misleading stories about bottled water not being any better than tap water because the bacteria count in bottled water is higher than that in tap water. These stories point out that there are no bacteria in tap water because of the chlorine. The problem is chlorine is a poison that kills living organisms. We, too, are living organisms. When we drink it, we're drinking poison. Yes, we're taking it in small amounts, but it's still a highly poisonous chemical and should not be consumed.

Chlorine has been shown to contribute to heart disease. It damages the arteries. People worry about cholesterol and focus on lowering it when it comes to heart disease, but cholesterol becomes a problem only when it attaches itself to the artery and then clogs it, restricting blood flow. And cholesterol only attaches itself to the artery when the artery is scarred or damaged.

Primarily, there are four things that cause the arteries to become scarred:

1. **Chlorinated water**. Chlorine in the water that you drink, shower and bathe in, or swim in causes scarring of the arteries, which in turn means no matter how much cholesterol you have or don't have, whatever cholesterol is there will attach itself and begin the clogging process.

2. **Hydrogenated oils or trans fats**. As you look at much of the processed food you buy in boxes, if you read the label you'll often see the words "hydrogenated oil" or "partially hydrogenated oil." These are trans fats. Margarine, for example, is a hydrogenated oil. These trans fats scar the arteries. They cause heart disease and arteriosclerosis.

3. **Homogenized dairy products**. People say, "Well I drink low-fat milk or low-fat yogurt." You're being misled. The fat isn't the problem. When dairy products are homogenized it turns them into a lethal man-made product that causes scarring of the arteries. It is not the fat that'll harm you, it's the homogenization process.

4. **Sugar**. In the last few years it's been discovered that sugar causes inflammation, which contributes to artery damage. A study published in the *Journal of The American College of Cardiology* found that consuming foods high in sugar led to a dysfunction in the layer of cells that line the arteries. Repeated sugar consumption reduces the flexibility of the arteries and leads to heart disease.

Okay, now let's get back to water. What kind of water do *I* drink? Never tap water. I have a reverse osmosis unit in my house. I have the water in my entire house filtered. I also have a distiller, which in addition to steam distillation, also gets rid of the energetic memory attached to the water. I *do* drink bottled water and spring water when I travel.

The reason I brought up the issue about arteriosclerosis is that tap water has chlorine in it. One reason there's so much heart disease today is because people not only drink tap water, they also bathe and shower in it, and swim in chlorinated pools. Since our skin is the largest organ in the body, it's believed that we absorb more chlorine and toxins by taking one shower than by drinking five glasses of water.

In a shower, not only is the chlorine being absorbed through the skin, the toxins are also turned into a gas created by the steam. These toxic fumes in your shower are then inhaled. Consider reducing this exposure by finding a good shower filtration system for your home, or better yet, a whole house filtration system.

Unfortunately, it's not just the water you drink and bathe in. Chlorine is used in the processing of many fruits and vegetables. It's also added to the water used in the irrigation of fruits and vegetables. Chlorine is a major problem.

As you can now understand, our water supply is loaded with toxins. These toxins are getting into our bodies by:

- ✔ Drinking the water

- ✔ Eating or drinking anything made with the water

- ✔ Eating any food that was grown with the water

- ✔ Eating any meat, poultry, fish or dairy where the animal drank the water

✔ Showering, bathing, or swimming in the water

Let's talk about other toxins you may put into your body via what you drink. How about carbonated sodas? Don't drink them. Carbonated beverages block calcium absorption. Calcium is one of the most important building blocks of nutrition. And have you read the ingredients in sodas? They're full of chemicals, plus high fructose corn syrup (which is a poison that makes you fat), and diet sodas are even worse. Artificial sweeteners in diets sodas are mostly, if not all, toxic.

What about alcohol? I mostly avoid it. I prefer to drink purified water and not much else, but sometimes a little wine (preferably red, because of its antioxidants) is okay.

Tea can be good and therapeutic. Choose organic blends.

What about juices? Be wary of store bought juice. It's processed. Unfortunately, when juice is processed, bacteria and mold can develop, which contaminates it. So by law the juice has to be pasteurized, which means it has to be heated to 220 degrees for thirty minutes to kill any bacteria so you don't get sick from it. This kills all of the living enzymes and destroys the natural energy of the fruit. The juice is then filtered, and in many cases, sugar (which isn't listed on the label) is added. It's not healthy, it's man-made, and it's tainted with chemicals and toxins. If you want juice, buy organic fruits and vegetables and juice them yourself at home.

> The things you apply to your skin get into your bloodstream as well.

Another way we absorb toxins is by applying them to our skin. Anything we put on the skin is absorbed into the body. This is why certain drugs (like hormones and nicotine patches) are administered through the skin. Those drugs pass through the skin and end up in the bloodstream. The things you apply to your skin get into your bloodstream as well.

Our friends at the FDA have determined that many chemicals are for "external use only." They're poisonous and cannot be taken internally because they can kill you. But remember, what you put on your body winds up in your body. Do you understand the problem here and why we take in so many toxins? We apply lotions, moisturizers, sunscreens, cosmetics, soap, shampoo, etc. Virtually all of these contain ingredients that even the FDA says are so poisonous that they can't be taken internally. Yet, they are deemed safe enough to be used on the skin. Be wary of this. Look at the products you use and consider making changes to natural products where you can.

For example, coconut oil makes an excellent moisturizer. Apple cider vinegar can be used as a skin toner. Baking soda can be used to brush your teeth and for deodorant. Underarm deodorants and antiperspirants contain chemicals that are believed to be a major cause of breast cancer. Remember, if you can't eat it, do not put it on your skin.

We also absorb toxins through the nose, via poisons in the air. Pollution is obviously a problem, but there are many toxins floating around that people are unaware of, or simply don't think about. Air fresheners are among the worst. Talk about misleading advertising. They claim that these products "freshen" the air, when actually they contain toxic chemicals. Would you consider opening the can and drinking the air freshener? Read the label since they even tell you how poisonous the ingredients are. These products eliminate odors by having you spray a poison in the air. This poison kills the receptors in the nose so that you can't smell the offending odor any more. Air fresheners don't eliminate odors; they eliminate your ability to smell them.

Other airborne toxins include: mold, dust, pollens, and the fumes emitted from carpeting, glue, paint, mattresses, laundry detergent, household cleaners etc. Any aroma that you smell means molecules are in the air and you're breathing them in. We're inhaling toxins on a regular basis. It's impossible to eliminate all of them. However, it is possible to reduce the number of toxins you're inhaling by avoiding commercial household products and using nontoxic products, or making your own. Baking soda, vinegar, and lemon can be used for all kinds of household cleaning, including laundry. An air purifier (with a filter, not an air *freshener*) reduces other airborne toxins.

It's important to note that what you inhale has an effect on such things as appetite, digestion, moods, depression, anxiety, irritability, and sleep. Reducing the toxins that you breathe can have a very profound impact on your health and wellbeing.

We also take in toxins **through our eyes.** The primary type of toxins that enter through the eyes are images that cause bad emotions. There are more violent images on television, in the movies, newspapers and magazines, video games, and books than ever before. Repeated exposure to negative, disturbing images causes the body to become acidic. Today, people are being exposed to over one thousand times the amount of negative images than they were just twenty years ago; and over ten thousand times the amount of negative images compared to seventy-five years ago. Be mindful of what you're watching, reading, and listening to. Too much negative stimulation is toxic and can lead to health problems.

Toxins get into our bodies **through the ears**, via anything we put into them, as well as the sounds we hear. Sounds are vibrations and frequencies. Certain vibrations and frequencies engender life. And other vibrations and frequencies can cause degeneration and death.

If we stop and really listen to all of the sounds around us, we find the majority are unnatural man-made frequencies. These frequencies go in through the ears and affect us right down to our cells. If the frequency is not in tune with what our bodies are equipped to tolerate, it can disrupt the natural balance of the body. The simplest proof of this is how certain music, sounds, and frequencies, can cause a plant to either die or thrive. Think of the opera singer who hits a high note and shatters a crystal glass. That is how powerful vibrations, sounds, and frequencies are. Sounds can affect the body in such a powerful way that even the U.S. military uses sound as a weapon that induces physiological and psychological damage.

Much of the noise we hear is beyond our control, but you should consider making changes to stressful sounds where you can. When you drive, you might listen to calm music rather than frenetic music, or the news. Alarm clocks are now using natural sounds, like waves, or rain to wake a person more gently. Earplugs or headphones can provide relief at times from stressful sounds. Just be mindful of negative sounds and noises and do what you can to minimize your exposure to them.

> Too much negative stimulation is toxic and can lead to health problems.

Now I'd like to you to consider a toxic cause of illness that people have only recently begun to be concerned about. That is electromagnetic fields. Medical science claims there is no evidence to prove that electromagnetic energy has an adverse effect on health. Remember, though, that science has also refuted things throughout history that have later proven to be true. Science claimed that there was no evidence that nutrition had an effect on health; or that cigarettes were addictive. Science stated that anyone believing those things were heretics. The same is true now in relation to electromagnetic energy. Think about it. If a satellite in the sky beams down electromagnetic energy twenty-four hours a day, seven days a week, and this energy is invisible, cannot be detected, yet has the ability to pass through almost any material, and contains so much information that a "receiver" converts it into the music of an orchestra or images on a TV screen, isn't it possible that this energy is also passing through our bodies? Is it possible that this unnatural energy could have a negative impact on our health? Here are a few examples of the sources of unnatural electromagnetic energy bombarding our bodies every day:

- ✔ **Satellites**. There are dozens of satellites beaming down unnatural electromagnetic energy twenty-four hours a day, seven days a week.

- ✔ **Radar**. Radar stations for national defense and weather emit harmful electromagnetic energy twenty-four hours a day, seven days a week. It's interesting to note that many people believe that when these radar stations are put on maximum power during times of heightened security, a higher percentage of people feel ill, fatigued, and depressed. There is also the suggestion that those living close to these powerful radar towers have a higher chance of getting cancer.

- ✔ **Cell phone towers.** These towers push out powerful energy waves on a consistent basis.

- ✔ **Cell phones**. When your cell phone is turned on it produces powerful unnatural electromagnetic energy, as well as drawing in all of the cell phone tower energy. If a cell phone is within just a few feet of you, you are being affected.

- ✔ **Wireless internet routers.** Wi-Fi modems use electromagnetic radiation to send their signals to your computer through walls, exposing you to radiation.

- ✔ **High-tension power lines.** These lines produce powerful amounts of negative energy affecting all living things in a large area around them.

- ✔ **Electric wiring**. Wiring encompasses our homes, our offices, our cars, any electronic device we carry, and is even buried under sidewalks and streets.

- ✔ **Computers, televisions and radios.** When these units are turned on, they emit large amounts of negative electromagnetic energy.

- ✔ **Fluorescent lights.** It is common knowledge that fluorescent lighting is an unnatural light source and can cause headaches, fatigue, and a weakening of the immune system. They also emit large doses of negative electromagnetic energy.

- ✔ **Microwave ovens**. The "microwaves" can be released from the oven adversely affecting those around it.

Another dynamic relating to electromagnetic energy is ions. There are positive and negative ions. Positively charged ions have an adverse effect on the body. Negatively charged ions have a positive, health-enhancing effect on the body. Running water such as a stream, waterfalls or the crashing waves of an ocean, emit large amounts of life-enhancing negative ions. The wind blowing through trees also emits these wonderful negative ions. This is why most people feel better when they're in these areas.

Conversely, the wind blowing through tall buildings in cities, or an electric dryer, emits harmful positive ions. If you sit in a Laundromat all day, it's common to feel horrible and fatigued. These harmful positive ions also can suppress your immune system.

Electromagnetic chaos can't be avoided altogether, however, you should try, where possible, to minimize your exposure to it. Turn off Wi-Fi modems at night. Minimize microwave usage. Don't hold your cell phone against your head or body (use a headset). And don't sleep with your cell phone turned on and right next to you. Avoid fluorescent lights. Don't leave televisions on around your house unnecessarily. Consider periodic detox days where you don't use any electronics.

What Comes Out of the Body

I've discussed toxins that are going *into* our bodies, but now let's talk about what goes *out* of the body. Our bodies produce toxins. This is fine, as long as the body's ability to eliminate these toxins is operating properly. Even if you put no toxins into your body, it would still create waste material and toxins. All toxins, whether created by the body or put into the body must be eliminated in order for us to be healthy. When toxins are allowed to accumulate they cause the immune system to be suppressed, and the body to become acidic. Accumulated toxins that have not been flushed out, or eliminated create an environment wherein illness and disease can flourish. We basically eliminate toxins through:

- ✔ The nose
- ✔ The mouth
- ✔ The urinary tract
- ✔ The colon
- ✔ The skin

The nose and mouth eliminate toxins primarily through the lungs. Our urinary tract eliminates toxins primarily through the kidneys and liver. The colon eliminates toxins primarily through the liver, the stomach and small intestine. The skin eliminates toxins primarily through perspiration.

Most people have excess accumulated toxins and waste in their bodies. The two main reasons for this are: 1) they're putting too many toxins into the body on a regular basis, and 2) their elimination channels are clogged, and/or sluggish.

When you take in toxins, and your body creates toxins at a faster rate than you're eliminating them, you build up an accumulation. For example, are your nasal and sinus cavities clear and mucus free? Do you breathe fully and deeply from your diaphragm, allowing your lungs to properly do their job? Do you sweat on a regular basis? Do you drink plenty of pure water, which allows the elimination channels to work more efficiently? Do you have bowel movements daily? A few common things that slow the elimination process are:

- ✔ **Antibiotics**. If you've ever taken an antibiotic you have dramatically slowed your elimination potential via the colon. Antibiotics kill all of the friendly bacteria in the intestine and colon. This allows unfriendly yeast, most notably Candida, to proliferate and infest your digestive system. This yeast overgrowth slows digestion, increases gas, bloating and constipation, and itself creates an abnormal number of toxins.

- ✔ **Lotions and creams.** Most people put lotions and creams all over their skin clogging the pores and suppressing the natural elimination process through the skin. This includes sunscreens, cosmetics, deodorants, and antiperspirants.

- ✔ **Lack of body movement**. Have you ever noticed when you take a dog for a walk, they poop? When you move your body as nature intended, you assist the elimination process. Since most people sit all day, their elimination cycles are suppressed. When you eat, food goes through the digestion process and ends up in the colon ready for elimination. The longer it sits in the colon, the more toxic it becomes. If left long enough, these toxins begin to enter the bloodstream. This can turn into a serious condition resulting in death. Your body's elimination system must be working at optimal levels if you want to live without illness and disease.

Exercise

In order to properly eliminate toxins you must exercise. In simplistic terms, there are seven kinds of exercise:

1. *Slow rhythmic movement.* This is mainly walking. The body is designed to walk, for long distances, and for long periods of time. Walking is probably the most important form of exercise you can do. When you go for a walk, not only are you getting the benefits of the slow rhythmic movement, your lymph system and digestive system are working toxins out of your body. The body is moving and energy is flowing through the meridians. Walking also has a profound effect on your state of mind and happiness factor.

2. *Stretching.* Your body consists of muscles, tendons, and ligaments. If you lived in a natural setting, interacting with nature as we are designed, the natural activities you would be doing throughout your day would cause the frequent stretching of your ligaments, muscles, and tendons. Lack of flexibility allows for negative energy and toxins to accumulate in parts of your body.

3. *Resistance exercise.* This includes any form of movement where resistance is put against a muscle, and the muscle is required to push or pull against the resistance. The most common form of resistance training is weight lifting or the use of resistance machines. Weight training can increase the size and strength of muscles, but it can reduce flexibility, thus hindering the flow of energy through the body. Nevertheless, doing any form of exercise is better than doing none at all.

4. *Postures.* Certain exercise regimes involve postures that are held for a period of time. The most commonly known is yoga. There are many forms of yoga. Not all are posture

based. Some yoga techniques are fluid and movement oriented. The benefits of postures are that they seem to help open up the natural energy channels in the body, and stimulate internal organs.

5. *Aerobic exercise.* Aerobic means "with air." Any form of exercise where you're breathing heavily but can still have a conversation is aerobic exercise. Aerobic exercise stimulates blood flow throughout the body, oxygenates the body and speeds the elimination of toxins.

6. *Anaerobic exercise.* Anaerobic means "without air." Any form of exercise where you are breathing so hard you can barely speak is anaerobic. The benefits are, generally, a tremendous stimulation to your entire system because, in effect, you are putting the survival of every cell in your body at risk because of the lack of oxygen. This is helpful in "reprogramming the body" and allowing it to increase the elimination of toxins and stop any cellular activity that's abnormal.

7. *Cellular exercise.* Jumping on a mini-trampoline, also known as a Rebounder, has been shown to stimulate and strengthen every cell in the body. This unique form of exercise dramatically increases the movement through the lymph system, stimulates every cell's elimination of toxins, and increases the strength and vitality of every cell in the body.

The major benefits of exercise include:

✔ **Increased oxygen to the cells**. Most people are deficient in the amount of oxygen they have in their bodies. Viruses and cancer, for example, cannot exist in an oxygen rich environment. An oxygen rich body is an alkaline body. An alkaline body is a body where disease and illness cannot exist.

✔ **Movement of lymph fluid**. The lymphatic system is an important element in the elimination process. Moving the body, as it was intended, increases the movement of lymph fluid, assisting with the elimination of toxins.

✔ **Cell stimulation**. Every cell in the body produces toxic waste. Every cell needs stimulation in order to eliminate its toxic waste and thrive normally. When a cell doesn't eliminate its toxic waste it can behave abnormally, which causes tumors, cancer, or the degeneration of vital organs in the body.

✔ **Opening of energy channels.** Energy flows through channels in the body. When these channels are blocked or congested, energy doesn't flow efficiently causing cell abnormalities and the suppression of the immune system, making the body susceptible to illness.

✔ **Releasing of tension and stress.** Stress is the silent killer. In simplistic terms, stress is holding on to negative energy. When negative energy is held, it can lodge itself into parts of the body.

Rest

Without proper rest, the cells are not given the opportunity to recharge and rejuvenate. Tired cells can't eliminate toxins efficiently. It's also during rest that most healing takes place. Most people don't get enough rest, and the rest they do get is not full and deep.

There are three elements of proper rest:

1. *The time in which you rest.* The most optimum time for the body to rest is when the sun is no longer shining. Ideally, a person would rest and sleep when the sun goes down and arise when the sun comes up. This is the natural cycle. However, most people's life styles do not allow this. Therefore they are resting and sleeping at non-optimal times. Each week a lunar cycle occurs starting at sundown every

Friday, ending at sundown every Saturday. This is absolutely the most ideal time for the body to recharge.

2. *The amount of hours you rest.* Although every person is unique, it appears that most operate better when getting eight hours of sleep. Studies show that people don't function as well if they receive fewer, or more, hours. The majority of people sleep fewer than eight hours, and then try to catch up by occasionally sleeping more. This does not allow optimal rejuvenation of the cells in your body.

3. *Rest and sleep should be deep.* Most people toss and turn at night.

Ideally you would not move for the entire sleep time. When sleep is full and deep, brainwave activity can occur, which stimulates the healing process throughout the body. A person who snores wakes up many times per night and unfortunately never reaches the deepest levels of sleep and so the body is never operating at optimal efficiency.

There's a difference between sleep and rest. The body can rest without going to sleep. Most people never take a "rest" during the day. The common pattern of waking up, working all day nonstop, going to bed late, never getting a full deep eight hours of peaceful sleep, results in a body that slowly begins to break down and never has a chance to heal and recharge. The body is very much like a battery. Like a battery, when the body's energy runs out, it must be recharged. If one did nothing else but get proper rest and sleep, that person's energy levels would skyrocket and they'd experience dramatically less illness and disease.

Thoughts

Thoughts are things. Your body is in fact a powerful electromagnetic transmitter and receiver of energy. Every thought you have can have a powerful impact on the cells in your body. Positive high vibrational thoughts can rid your body of disease. Negative stressful low vibrational thoughts can *give* your body disease.

Science tends not to believe that thoughts can have a profound effect on health. However, it is interesting to point out that medical science can't dispute the "placebo" effect. The placebo effect is when a person is given a "placebo," like a sugar pill, yet their disease is cured. This occurs because the patient thinks that what he or she is taking will cure the disease. This happens in as many as 40 percent of cases. Imagine, up to 40 percent of the time a person with a dreaded disease is cured with his or her own thoughts! Yet, remember our friends at the FDA insist that only a drug can cure disease.

Thoughts can heal, but they can also cause sickness and disease. Stress, which could be defined as negative thoughts, causes the body to become acidic, thus creating an environment for illness and disease. These negative thoughts can be conscious or unconscious. Worrying about money, arguing with relatives, friends, and co-workers, watching scary movies and reading the news, all increase stress levels.

> Thoughts can heal, but they can also cause sickness and disease.

Many negative thoughts are trapped in stressful or traumatic incidences from our past. Several doctors have found that the majority of people with cancer have an incident in their past that caused tremendous grief. Individuals who have heart attacks are found to have suppressed anger. It's interesting to note the correlation between emotions and certain diseases. The good news is this can be reversed.

Author Earl Nightingale discovered what he called "the strangest secret": *You become what you think about.* Positive thoughts and low amounts of stress create an alkaline pH in the body, wherein we don't become ill. Negative thoughts and emotions, and high levels of stress cause the body to become acidic, leading to illness and disease.

What You Say

Words have power. Most people speak words that increase stress and turn the body's pH from alkaline to acidic. Words can change the way we think and feel. Researchers have concluded that speaking the correct form of words and thinking the correct thoughts change a person's DNA.

Of all the things I've talked about in this chapter thus far relating to why we get sick, please do not overlook the power of how you think, and what you say. These two factors dramatically contribute to stress levels. Stress absolutely causes illness and disease. Reducing stress is one of the most powerful natural cures for virtually every disease in the body. This is one of those cures that can't be patented. No one's going to make billions of dollars selling it to you, but simple stress reducing techniques that are effective and inexpensive have been proven to be one of the most powerful natural cures of all time. This is one of the "natural cures" that "they" don't want you to know about.

The conclusion, then, is that we get sick because: We're putting too many toxins in our body and not flushing them out fast enough. We are not putting enough of the necessary nutrients into our body, and the nutrients that *are* going in are not being properly absorbed. We are exposed to, and negatively affected by electromagnetic chaos. And we have trapped mental and emotional stress.

Since all matter consists ultimately of energy, in simplistic terms, the cause of all disease is energetic imbalance.

CHAPTER 6

How To Never Get Sick Again

This chapter will give you the information to help you eliminate any illness or disease and prevent any illness and disease in the future. This information will also allow you to potentially slow down or even reverse the aging process. Keep in mind that this information is my opinion and based on the information currently available.

Right now, you either have some known illness or disease such as cancer, diabetes, etc., or you claim to be healthy. If you claim to be healthy, you probably still experience the occasional aches and pains, fatigue, headaches, indigestion, colds and flu, heartburn, etc. So-called healthy people believe that these occasional conditions are "normal." They are not. A healthy person has little, if any, body odor, no bad breath, no foot odor, their urine and stool don't smell bad, they sleep soundly, they have no skin rashes or dandruff, they're not depressed or stressed and they don't get aches and pains, or colds and flu. Truly healthy people are full of energy and vitality, and never have to take any nonprescription or prescription drug because they never have any symptoms that require medication.

It is hard to find a truly healthy person. Let's examine where you are right now. Most likely, you're full of toxins. You're also probably deficient in necessary nutrients. The energy in your body is not flowing properly. Many of your systems are not operating at optimal levels. You either notice severe symptoms, or you have mild symptoms that you classify as normal.

What can we do to (a) eradicate any and all symptoms you have, thus "curing" the disease or illness and (b) prevent any illness or disease from starting, thus giving you a boost in energy, vitality, and vibrant health?

In general terms, the way to eradicate any illness and disease you may have, prevent illness and disease from occurring in the future, and slow down or potentially reverse the aging process is to do the following:

1. Eliminate the toxins that have built up in your system. You're loaded with toxins. The only question is, how much? You must get these toxins out of your body if you want to cure and prevent illness and disease. Getting the toxins out of your body can immediately increase energy, help you lose weight, eliminate depression and anxiety, and potentially reverse most illnesses and disease. The basic cleanses that you should do are:
    (a) colon cleanse
    (b) liver/gallbladder cleanse
    (c) kidney/bladder cleanse
    (d) heavy metal cleanse
    (e) parasite cleanse
    (f) Candida cleanse
    (g) full-body fat tissue/lymphatic cleanse

A simple Internet search will lead you to options for the aforementioned cleanses.

2. Stop, or at least reduce, the toxins entering your body. It's impossible to totally eliminate toxins from entering your body, but you can dramatically reduce the amount of toxins going in.

3. Make sure your elimination systems are clean and not sluggish, thus allowing the toxins that you do put in your body, and the toxins that develop naturally are getting eliminated quickly and not accumulating.

4. Make sure you're getting proper nutrition in the form of vitamins, minerals, enzymes, cofactors, and life-sustaining "energy," and make sure your system can assimilate these nutrients.

5. Reduce and/or neutralize the electromagnetic energy that is attacking your body's energy field and cells.

6. Reduce stress.

7. Use your mind and words to create a healthy alkaline body pH, and actually change genetically defective DNA structures into healthy DNA structures.

Theoretically, if all of the above were to occur you couldn't get sick. If the cause of all disease is too many toxins, nutritional deficiencies, electromagnetic chaos, and/or stress, then if you did not have toxins in the body, if you did not have nutritional deficiencies, if you did not have exposure to electromagnetic chaos, and if you did not have stress, then you would not have any disease.

I'm going to list many things for you to consider doing that will help you accomplish the recommendations above. Do not be overwhelmed by this list. Don't think that you must do all of these things starting tomorrow if you want to prevent and cure any disease you have. Consider going at an easy pace, and implementing these things slowly and in a way that's comfortable for you. If you do these things, in my opinion, you virtually should never get sick. If you do get sick, the severity and duration of the illness will be short.

> You can help the body heal better and faster, but you can't heal the body.

Remember, the body heals itself. No treatment heals or cures. You can help the body heal better and faster, but you can't heal the body. All of the suggestions in this chapter are designed to help the body heal itself. All of these suggestions are designed to turn your body's pH from acidic, where disease and illness can develop, to the healthy state of alkaline, where disease and illness cannot exist. There is no *one* thing that can turn your body from acidic pH to alkaline pH. It depends upon what's *causing* your body to be acidic and that could be a number of things. But if you do the things in this chapter, your body *can* turn from acidic to alkaline pH. That's one of our ultimate goals and it's one of the simplest ways to determine how healthy you are. If your body's pH is alkaline, it is virtually impossible to get cancer or any other major disease.

Here are what I believe to be the simple all natural, non-drug and nonsurgical ways to prevent and cure every disease.

1. **See a natural healthcare provider on a regular basis.**

   Choose one that doesn't only use drugs or surgery. When you have a car that you love and cherish, you keep it clean on the inside and out. You do not wait for the car to make funny noises or stop running; instead you bring the car in for regular maintenance. This maintenance is designed to prevent major problems from occurring. Your body should be treated in a similar manner. You should be seeing various natural healthcare providers from a variety of disciplines, even when you aren't experiencing symptoms. I believe it's important to be looked at by several people and get multiple opinions. Even though I feel I'm knowledgeable when it comes to the prevention and curing of disease naturally, I also know that getting other perspectives is valuable. Avoid being seen or treated by a doctor who uses drugs and surgery. Choose a licensed healthcare practitioner. Some examples I highly recommend are:

a. Get treated by a bioenergetic synchronization technique practitioner.

Dr. M.T. Morter, Jr., who invented the technique, has trained thousands of people in this treatment. It's painless and takes only a few minutes, and it effectively rebalances the body, reducing or eliminating pain or trauma. It helps the body go from acid to alkaline. For more information, go to www.morterhealth.com.

b. Get a chiropractic adjustment.

If you've never had a chiropractic adjustment, you probably need one. Because of our lifestyle, our spines get misaligned. Realigning the spine allows energy to flow freely throughout the body. I see several different chiropractors, because each has a different style of treatment, and I visit one at least once a month for a tune-up. Even if you have no pain, go get an adjustment. The adjustments are painless and most people feel energized afterwards.

c. See an herbalist.

Seeing a highly-recommended herbalist allows you to be treated effectively, and yet avoid the dangers of drugs. If you've never had a consultation with an herbalist you have no idea what you're missing. When you take in herbs specifically customized for you, the physical benefits can be enormous.

d. See a homeopathic practitioner.

Homeopathy is a system of treatment in which homeopathic medicines are used to gently bring the body into balance. A good homeopathic doctor does not treat symptoms, but instead, treats the whole person.

e. See a naturopath.

Naturopaths are licensed healthcare practitioners who differ from homeopaths in that they may prescribe *multiple* types of treatment (herbs, supplements, dietary adjustment), yet no prescription drugs or surgery. They use a holistic approach to bring a person to a state of balance, thus allowing the body to cure itself.

2. Stop taking nonprescription and prescription drugs.

If you're taking drugs of any kind, do not do this step without consulting your physician. Remember, drugs are poisons. This includes vaccines. Although opinions vary, many experts believe that vaccines are some of the most toxic substances you can put in your body. It is estimated that millions have had to receive medical treatment because of horrible side effects from taking prescription and nonprescription drugs. It's also estimated that tens of millions will develop long-term medical conditions because they took nonprescription and prescription drugs. In my opinion, drugs should only be taken in the most severe cases. This step is so important. You have to know that if you are taking any nonprescription or prescription drugs you absolutely will get sick and develop disease. Let me say that again: If you continue to take nonprescription over-thecounter drugs and/or prescription drugs you absolutely will get sick. Nonprescription drugs and prescription drugs are toxins and they *cause* illness and disease. You must stop taking them if you intend to prevent and cure any disease. You cannot cure your disease if you continue to take nonprescription and prescription drugs. You cannot prevent disease if you continue to take nonprescription and prescription drugs. In my opinion, you should clean out your medicine cabinet and stop giving your money to the criminals who run the drug companies.

3. **Energetic rebalancing.**

    Frequency generators have been around for decades. Today there are several machines using frequencies to balance a person's energy, thus eliminating the energetic frequency of the imbalance or disease. When the frequency of the disease you have has been neutralized, the disease goes away. These machines allow the body to cure all diseases. They're fast, painless, and inexpensive, and they are also outlawed by the FDA. Individual practitioners using these machines never publicly claim that they cure anything for fear that the FDA will prosecute them for using an unlicensed medical device and curing people without the legally approved drugs. These machines include the Intero, Vegatest, Dermatron, and others. I've been using this technology for several years, and I have never in that time been sick. When everyone around me got the flu, I never experienced a symptom.

    People always want to know what the "natural cure" is for their disease, or what the best way to prevent disease is. If you do the three things I have just mentioned— (1) see several licensed health-care practitioners for individualized treatment; (2) stop taking all nonprescription over-the-counter drugs and prescription drugs (under the supervision of a doctor); and (3) get on an energetic rebalancing program, I believe you will virtually never get sick and you can cure any disease you have, provided you're not past the point of no return. If you *are* past the point of no return and the degeneration or disease is in its most advanced stages, then unfortunately it's too late to implement these cures.

Can energetic rebalancing alone prevent and cure all disease? I believe that it can. I've seen this technology cure people of the most horrific debilitating diseases anyone can imagine. I have seen cancer, diabetes, MS and countless other diseases cured by energetic rebalancing. The thousands of people who are on energetic rebalancing technology virtually never get sick. This is statistically unheard of. However, the FDA, other government agencies, and all of the groups I mentioned previously categorically do not want this technology exposed and they try to debunk it and attack it every chance they can. Why? Because it will cost them billions of dollars in profits if people use this inexpensive technology to prevent and cure their diseases. You can go to the Internet to find various energetic rebalancing treatments. I am on two programs. One is available at www.energeticbalancing.us and www.energeticmatrix.com.

4. **Check your body pH.**

Dr. M.T. Morter (whom I mentioned earlier in the chapter) discovered one of the greatest breakthroughs for health assessment in the last hundred years, yet because this discovery would not increase profits to the pharmaceutical industry it has gone by the wayside without much fanfare. Dr. Morter's discovery should have won him a Nobel Prize. He discovered the powerful truth that when your body's pH is acidic, diseases such as cancer, diabetes, and Multiple Sclerosis can thrive. He also discovered that when a body's pH is alkaline, diseases such as cancer cannot exist. Therefore, one of the most powerful and simplest ways to test your health and/or propensity for disease is to check your body's pH.

The pH testing procedure is something I encourage everyone to do on a regular basis. I check mine monthly. If it's out of the proper range I look at the things I'm doing, or not doing, and I can make simple adjustments to correct the out of balance pH. The reason this is so important is because it takes years to develop most diseases. When you're checking your pH regularly, even if it goes out of balance, as long as you correct it and bring it back into balance, you are never allowing your body the time to develop a disease. In my opinion it's the simplest and easiest way to make sure you never develop any major illnesses.

The above four suggestions are what I call the basic four for the prevention and treatment of all disease. In my opinion, you must do these if you're serious about achieving and maintaining optimal health. However, we know that the causes of all disease are (1) too many toxins in the body, (2) nutritional deficiencies, (3) electromagnetic chaos, and (4) stress. Therefore, we must address each of these with specific recommendations on how to achieve (a) no toxins in the body, (b) no nutritional deficiencies, (c) no electromagnetic chaos, and (d) no stress.

Here are the specific recommendations. Doing these things will turn your body's pH from acid to alkaline and create a state of balance in the body known as *homeostasis*.

A. Clean Out The Toxins That Have Accumulated In Your Body.

It's important to understand that from the time you're born your body is flooded with toxins. These include everything from vaccines, to nonprescription and prescription drugs, the air you breathe, the water you drink as well as shower, bathe and swim in, and all of the chemicals put in your food. They also include all of the toxins from carpeting, paint, non-stick cookware, cosmetics, makeup, soaps, lotions, and sunscreens. For years, your body has been loaded with toxins and these toxins don't fully leave the body. They stay in the fatty tissues; they stay in the organs; they stay in the colon, intestine and throughout your entire body. They are causing you illness and disease. They're suppressing your immune system. If you want to prevent disease you must clean these toxins out.

If you want to prevent disease you must clean these toxins out.

If the toxins in our bodies are the *cause* of the illnesses and diseases that we're suffering from, then if we clean the toxins out of our bodies, *in most cases*, we'll experience a dramatic reduction, or even a complete elimination, of our symptoms. Simply cleaning toxins out of your body could be the "natural cure" of your disease.

Keep in mind, if you're experiencing symptoms or have a disease, it may have taken years to develop that illness. If you clear out all of the toxins in your system it may take several months after that for the body to heal itself. Do give it some time. This is why, again, I encourage you to be under the care of a licensed healthcare practitioner.

Here are the best ways to clean the toxins out of your system:

1. **Get fifteen colonics in thirty days.**
   Right now as you read this there's an excellent chance that you have several pounds of undigested fecal matter in your colon. This waste matter is suppressing your immune system, potentially causing gas, bloating and constipation, dramatically reducing the assimilation of nutrients, and slowing

your metabolism. Getting a series of fifteen colonics over a thirty-day period is one of the most important first steps in cleansing and detoxifying your body. Most people lose between three and fifteen pounds simply by doing this procedure. The hair, skin, and nails begin to radiate and glow with health. Your energy levels can sky rocket, depression, stress, anxiety and fatigue are usually dramatically reduced or eliminated. Food cravings are reduced or vanish completely.

2. **Do a colon cleanse.**
   If you do the colonics, you won't need a colon cleanse as well. But a clean colon is an important step in ridding your body of accumulated toxins.

3. **Do a liver/gallbladder cleanse.**
   This cleanse generally causes the removal of gallstones that contain accumulated toxins and which people are usually unaware that they have. As a result of their removal, the liver will function more efficiently and when it does, the liver itself removes toxins from the body.

4. **Do a kidney/bladder cleanse.**
   Cleansing the kidney and bladder will help these organs function more efficiently. The kidneys and bladder are filters in the body and when they're sluggish due to toxic build up, it only leans to more toxic accumulation.

5. **Do a heavy metal cleanse.**
   Exposure to heavy metals can create all kinds of problems. Some of these heavy metals can affect the brain. In some cases, heavy metal toxicity leads to Multiple Sclerosis.

6. **Do a parasite cleanse.**
   Parasites, like heavy metals, are a major cause of disease. There are different types of parasites and they affect different parts of the body. Common types are in the intestines and they can prevent the body from absorbing nutrients.

7. **Do a Candida cleanse.**

   If you've ever taken antibiotics any time in your life, you likely have a Candida yeast overgrowth. This overgrowth is most common in the intestine, but it can infiltrate your entire body. This overgrowth can be a cause of virtually every symptom you can imagine: headaches, gas bloating, indigestion, heartburn, nausea, allergies, asthma, fibromyalgia, arthritis, diabetes, constipation, yeast infections, dandruff, acne, bad breath, fatigue, depression, stress, and on and on. Doing a program that eliminates Candida from your body is one of the backbones of good health. The most common side effect of excess Candida is the inability to lose weight. People who eliminate Candida tend to lose weight without trying. Candida also causes food cravings and can make you eat when you're not hungry. When Candida is normalized, a person's appetite can be dramatically reduced.

8. **Do a full-body fat/lymphatic cleanse.**

   The lymph system—the lymph nodes and vessels absorb excess fluid and debris from our bodies. When that system gets congested it leads to problems. Cleansing the lymph system includes dietary changes, dry-brushing, massage and exercise, all of which assist the body in moving fluid through the lymph system. This is necessary, because the lymph system doesn't have a pump the way the circulatory system has the heart.

9. **Drink eight glasses of pure water daily.**

   As I've mentioned previously all tap water is toxic because it contains chlorine. Most tap water also has fluoride, which is one of the most poisonous and disease causing agents you can put in your body. Do not drink or use tap water for any reason except for washing your floor. You need to drink water, though, and the water must be pure. Water is instrumental not only in flushing and nourishing the body, but also in keeping it hydrated and pH balanced. I recommend drinking a minimum of eight large glasses of water daily. Use a water purifier or bottled spring water.

10. **Use a rebounder (mini-trampoline) ten minutes a day.**

    A rebounder is a mini-trampoline. Using this device for just ten minutes a day can provide more cellular benefit than almost any other form of exercise. A rebounder stimulates every cell in the body simultaneously. It strengthens the immune system and it's effective at purging toxins from the cells. It stimulates all major organs and glands, and dramatically strengthens and tones the muscles, tendons, and ligaments. A truly spectacular form of exercise.

11. **Walk one hour a day.**

    The body is designed to walk. Walking outside reduces stress, stimulates the lymphatic system, promotes a lean body, and helps alleviate depression.

12. **Stretch the muscles and tendons.**

    If your body is supple and flexible, energy easily flows and blockages do not occur. When energy flows it's less likely for illness and disease to manifest. I recommend doing yoga, Pilates, martial arts, or any other kind of exercise that leads to stretching on a regular basis. I spend fifteen minutes each morning stretching.

13. **Practice deep breathing.**

    Your lungs need to be used. Most Americans breathe from high up in their chests. If you watch babies breathe naturally, you'll notice that they breathe fully and deeply. Their stomachs and diaphragms expand as well as their chests and backs. Deep breathing everyday stimulates the immune system, increases metabolism, reduces stress, and brings vital oxygen into the body. Most people are oxygen deficient.

Increasing oxygen to the cells can eliminate a multitude of diseases. Cancer, for example, cannot live in an oxygen-rich environment.

14. **Sweat with a regular dry sauna or an infrared sauna (not a wet steam).**
    Your body is supposed to sweat. It is a natural way to eliminate toxins. If you don't sweat, toxins build up in the system.

15. **Do oil pulling regularly.**
    Oil pulling is when you take a teaspoon or two of oil, generally extra virgin coconut oil, or castor oil, and swish it through the teeth as you would mouthwash. Do this for a few minutes or longer, up to 15 minutes. Coconut oil and castor oil are antibacterial and oil pulling with them will remove bacteria and toxins from parts of your mouth and from between the teeth. Did you know that there's a relationship between oral health and heart health? While the plaque in arteries is not the same as the plaque in between our teeth, there is a link. Bacteria from the mouth can enter the bloodstream through the gums and that same bacteria has been found clumped in artery plaque. Oil pulling removes the toxins and bacteria.

16. **Dry brush massage.**
    I mentioned dry-brushing earlier; it assists the lymphatic system. Dry-brushing also exfoliates the skin, and helps rid the body of toxins.

17. **Get a full-body Swedish and/or deep tissue massage on a regular basis.**
    The benefits of massage are reflected in your ...

    Circulatory System by:
    - helping to develop a stronger heart
    - improving oxygen supply to cells
    - improving the supply of nutrients to cells
    - eliminating metabolic wastes

- decreasing blood pressure
- increasing circulation of lymph nodes

Digestive System by:
- relaxing the abdominal and intestinal muscles
- relieving tension
- stimulating activity of liver and kidneys
- eliminating waste material

Muscular System by:
- relaxing or stimulating muscles
- strengthening muscles and connective tissue
- helping to keep muscles flexible and pliable
- relieving soreness, tension, and stiffness

Nervous System by:
- stimulating motor nerve points
- relieving restlessness and insomnia
- promoting a sense of well-being
- relieving pain

Respiratory System by:
- developing respiratory muscles
- draining sluggish lymph nodes

Lymphatic System by:
- cleansing the body of metabolic wastes
- draining sluggish lymph nodes

Integumentary System (the skin) by:
- stimulating blood to better nourish skin
- improving tone and elasticity of skin
- helping to normalize glandular functions

Skeletal System by:
- improving body alignment
- relieving stiff joints
- relieving tired aching feet

There are many kinds of massages. You may like one and not the other. I get at least one massage a week. They're highly therapeutic, and I recommend you get as many as you can as often as you can. Use different massage therapists to experience the full range of treatments.

18. **Do Chi Kung.**

Chi Kung is a series of gentle movements that stimulate strength, energy flow, increased energy, and many other health benefits. I have a friend named Peter Ragnar who lives in Tennessee and is a senior citizen. He has the body and skin of an athlete in his thirties. No one would ever guess this man's age. He practices most of the concepts described in this book. One of the things he does, which he believes is a major cause of his youthful appearance and incredible health, is Chi Kung ten minutes a day. Because the Earth's magnetic energy is so much lower today than it was thousands of years ago, he does the simple movements standing on powerful magnets. This technique is very effective. People who practice Chi Kung usually feel a major increase in physical energy within just a few days. Sleeping is improved and people report an increased sense of peace and wellbeing.

19. **Do Tai Chi.**

Tai Chi is a series of flowing movements designed to center oneself, relieve stress, increase energy flow, increase flexibility and strength, and promote health and wellbeing. I've practiced Tai Chi for over twenty years. There are many different teachers, some better than others, but doing any form of Tai Chi has benefits.

20. **Do a seven to thirty day fast.**

Fasting has numerous benefits, including giving the digestive system a rest so it can heal itself. It also helps rid the body of toxins. Doing a fast can help to reset your eating habits as well. After a fast you are less likely to crave unhealthy food and so you may have an easier time implementing healthy eating habits. Make sure to be under the supervision of a healthcare practitioner if you undertake a fast that's longer than a week.

21. **Get "specialized treatments" as needed.**
    Treatments such as reflexology, acupuncture, cranial sacral therapy, reiki, essential oil treatments, and various other holistic, all natural therapies have profound positive effects on health.

Obviously, when a person looks at this list their initial reaction is to be overwhelmed. You may feel there's no way you can do all of these things. That's okay. Start with doing *something*. You'll notice the first thing that I listed was doing fifteen colonics in thirty days. Start with that one. You'll feel more energetic than ever before. Just cleaning the colon, in the vast majority of cases, has been known to cure many diseases.

Each one of the things mentioned above is in fact a "natural cure" that "they" don't want you to know about. They're natural, they're not patentable, nobody's making billions of dollars on them, *and* they expose the fact that the drug industry and the food industry are causing the majority of illness and disease by feeding us chemical poisons. This is a fact that the powers that be don't want you to know, but the fact is indisputable.

B. You Must Stop Putting Toxins into the Body

I just gave you a list of things to do to get toxins *out* of the body. It's important now to reduce the amount of toxins going *into* the body on an ongoing basis. The recommendations that follow will dramatically reduce the amount of toxins you're putting in your body. Keep in mind that all of the recommendations in this chapter have a profound effect on preventing and curing disease, because they're addressing the cause of the symptoms and disease. They also have a profound effect upon changing your body's pH from acidic to alkaline.

Medical science does not want you to know what's causing your disease; they only want to sell you drugs to suppress the symptoms. Imagine a guy who says, "Every time I pour gasoline all over my house and light it with a match it burns to the ground. What's the cure?" You'd laugh at such a ridiculous statement, but that's what people do every day in relation to their own diseases. They don't realize that they're causing the disease with the toxins they put in their bodies.

...symptoms didn't develop overnight, and if you stop putting the toxins in, the symptoms are not necessarily going to vanish overnight...

A question that comes up is which of these is more important, or which will have the most profound affect. The answer is every person is different; however, generally speaking, the more powerful techniques are at the top of each list. Sometimes just making one change can eradicate your symptoms. You must keep in mind that your symptoms didn't develop overnight, and if you stop putting the toxins in, the symptoms are not necessarily going to vanish overnight either, although in some cases they do. Generally, it takes weeks or months for the symptoms to slowly diminish unless, as I mentioned, you're at the point of no return.

With that in mind, here is a powerful list of things to do and things *not* to do that will reduce the deadly poisons from going into your body and allow you to prevent and cure illness and disease.

1. **Do not eat any food that's produced or sold by a publicly traded corporation or that is a "brand name" product.**
   This is a tough one. If it comes in any mass produced packaging, then it came from a mass production processing plant. If you have ever been in a mass production food processing facility, you would understand what I'm talking about. Remember that there are over 15,000 chemicals that are routinely put into the food in the processing cycle that do not have to be listed on the label. Even if you read the ingredient list, there's an excellent chance that the food itself has been produced with chemicals and chemicals have been added. So, virtually all food you buy at the supermarket that comes in a package is loaded with chemicals. Mass produced food in packages is categorically unhealthy. If you must buy something in a box, jar, can, or package, buy something that was produced by hand in a small facility and look for the words "100% organic."

2. **Get the metal out of your dental work.**
   It's important for you to know that many people suffer horrible, debilitating symptoms that are *directly caused* by the amalgam (metal) fillings in their dental work. People have seen Multiple Sclerosis symptoms subside after removing these fillings, which generally are 50% mercury. Mercury is a powerful neurotoxin and it can cause neurological problems, mental disorders, chronic illnesses and autoimmune disease. If you currently have metal fillings, see a dentist who can replace them with nontoxic, nonmetal ones.

3. **Stop smoking.**
   This one is patently obvious. Not only should you not smoke, you should not allow anyone to smoke anywhere near you, either. Smoking is a horrible, toxic practice that causes and contributes to countless illnesses. Presumably, if you're interested enough in this book to be reading it,

you have the good sense not to smoke. But if you've been unable to quit, you must. Don't use the products made by the pharmaceutical industry. Those, too, are toxins. If you're struggling to quit, consider seeing a hypnotherapist. Many people also find acupuncture helpful.

4. **Don't drink tap water.**

All tap water is loaded with contaminants, toxins, poisons, and known cancer causing agents including fluoride and chlorine. Drinking tap water causes illness and disease.

But you must drink lots of water. However, the water has to be *pure*. Bottled spring water, water filtered using reverse-osmosis, and water purified through steam distillation, are all better options than tap water.

5. **Use a shower filter.**

Your skin absorbs the water from your shower or bath. A hot shower produces steam and that turns many of the chemicals in the water into poisonous gases. These gases are inhaled or absorbed through the skin. A good shower filter removes most of the toxins in the water.

6. **Eat only 100% organic food.**

You want to eat food that has not been grown with chemical fertilizers, pesticides, or herbicides. Organic food has no chemical poison residue, and has higher concentrations of nutrients.

7. **Do not eat in fast food restaurants.**

Fast food is simply some of the most nutritionally deficient and chemically loaded "food" on the planet. If the definition of food was "fuel for the body that also encourages life," fast food could no longer be called food. "Fast, good tasting *poison*," is a more accurate description. Oh, and did I tell you that it's designed to increase your appetite, and make you physically addicted to it. If you eat fifteen meals per week in a fast food restaurant, you have a 90 percent chance of getting cancer, heart disease, diabetes, acid reflux, obesity, and potentially dozens of other diseases. Avoid it completely.

8. **Never microwave food in plastic containers.**
   I don't use microwaves myself, because I believe it compromises the food by making it energetically toxic to the body, but others disagree. I also believe that being exposed to "microwaves" on a regular basis exposes you to toxins, so I would recommend that you avoid them. But I also understand that may be difficult for many people. If you are going to microwave your food, at least don't use plastic containers when you do it. Use a glass or ceramic, microwave safe dish. When you microwave certain plastics, a chemical called bisphenol A (BPA) can leach out of the plastic and migrate into the food making it toxic.

9. **Eliminate aspartame and monosodium glutamate.**
   Aspartame, aka NutraSweet®, is responsible for many distressing medical problems, ranging from headaches and memory loss, to hyperactivity in children, and seizure disorders. Both monosodium glutamate (MSG) and aspartame can cause harm to the brain and nervous system, and both have been linked to Alzheimer's disease, Lou Gehrig's disease, depression, Multiple Sclerosis, and more. MSG is a major cause of treatable and preventable illnesses such as headaches, asthma, epilepsy, heart irregularities, depression, and attention deficit/hyperactivity disorder.

10. **Do not eat artificial sweeteners (including Splenda).**
    Artificial sweeteners are man-made chemicals. They are poisons and should never be consumed. They cause all kinds of health problems. Instead, use raw organic honey, or coconut sugar, both of which have a lower glycemic index than regular sugar, or use the herb stevia, which comes from a plant.

11. **Do not eat processed sugar.**

There's been a lot written about the dangers of sugar in the past few years. Dr. Robert Lustig, an endocrinologist now famous for his lecture "Sugar: The Bitter Truth," which was written about in the New York Times, has even deemed sugar toxic, and many agree with him. The spike in blood sugar caused by ingesting all types of sugar is apparently worse for the body than previously believed. Sugar causes inflammation. Inflammation is detrimental to the immune system. In addition to leading to obesity and diabetes, new evidence suggests that sugar consumption can also cause damage to the arteries, contributing to heart disease. Minimize your sugar consumption and never eat white sugar. I recommend raw organic honey or coconut sugar in small amounts, or stevia.

12. **Do not drink sodas.**

All sodas are laden with chemical additives and all carbonated soft drinks block calcium absorption. Regular sodas are loaded with sugar. And did you know that Coke contains enough acid it can be used as rust remover? If it does that, what do think it's doing inside your body? *Nothing good,* that's what! Diet sodas have been called the "new crack" because they're so addictive. The artificial sweeteners in diet sodas can actually make you gain weight, because they stimulate the appetite, but they don't satisfy it. Studies have shown that consumption of diet sodas raised blood sugar levels.

13. **Do not eat hydrogenated oil.**

This is classified as a trans fat. Hydrogenated oils are man-made products. They are toxic. More importantly, they attack the artery walls and contribute to heart disease. They also attack the liver, spleen, intestine, kidneys, and gallbladder, causing these internal organs to operate much less efficiently. The bad news is that hydrogenated oil is in virtually every product you buy at the grocery store. The good news is that if you shop at a health food or whole food store, and if you read the labels, you can find many products without hydrogenated oil. This is a good example of how medical science says something is bad, and then later reverses its position. For years heart patients were told to stay away from butter because it was bad for your heart. They were told to use margarine instead. Margarine contains trans fat. Now we hear from the same medical community that margarine is in fact, much worse than butter. Avoid trans fats.

14. **Do not eat homogenized and pasteurized dairy products.**
All dairy products are not created equal. Raw milk that hasn't been pasteurized or homogenized, that came from a cow that was organically raised, was free-roaming, grass fed and not given antibiotics or growth hormone injections, will affect the body much differently (and better) than pasteurized and homogenized milk coming from a genetically modified cow that has been given antibiotics and growth hormone injections, never been allowed to roam, and has been fed chemically laced growth enhancing feed. Homogenization causes milk and other dairy products to be detrimental to the arteries and thus contribute to heart disease. Standard supermarket varieties of milk and dairy products are unhealthy. Organic raw, unpasteurized, non-homogenized milk, cheese and dairy products are beneficial.

15. **Do not eat high fructose corn syrup.**
High fructose corn syrup (HFCS) is used primarily for two reasons. First, it is inexpensive. Secondly, it makes you fatter than other sweeteners. The food industry wants you to be fat. Fat people eat more food, thus increasing sales and profits for the food companies. HFCS contributes to

fat deposits in your liver increasing buildup of lipoproteins. It also leads to plaque build-up in your arteries. Consuming it increases the likelihood of diabetes. And, studies have linked mercury with HFCS. As I've mentioned, mercury can cause neurological problems including Multiple Sclerosis. Never eat anything that contains high fructose corn syrup. Nearly *all* processed foods in the grocery store: catsup, relish, barbecue sauce, ice cream, cookies, canned fruit, lunch meats, juices, peanut butter and more contain this poison. If you're currently eating things that contain HFCS and you stop, you'll find that you lose weight. You'll also be at less risk for disease.

16. **Do not use fluoride toothpaste.**

Fluoride is a poison. Its supposed benefits to teeth have been largely overstated. Many studies have challenged the efficacy of fluoride to protect against tooth decay. And yet, it continues to be used as a selling point for toothpaste. Don't buy into that. You do not need fluoride and it is not good for you. Fluoride has been shown to increase absorption of aluminum, which can contribute to Alzheimer's disease. Fluoride has been linked to osteoporosis and bone cancer. You can find non-fluoridated toothpastes online or in a health food store. A paste made with baking soda and coconut oil works well, too.

17. **Do not use nonstick cookware.**

When nonstick cookware is heated to high temperatures it emits toxic fumes that can kill a small bird if it's close enough! These fumes, when inhaled by humans, lead to respiratory disease, weakening of the immune system, cancer, depression, asthma, headaches, and a multitude of other health problems.

18. **Eat only organic, kosher meat and poultry.**

Any meat or poultry that's not organic and kosher is highly toxic. Generally speaking:

o A conventional animal is injected with growth hormones and antibiotics, meaning that the meat we consume is then loaded with these drugs.

o A conventional animal is not allowed to roam freely or exercise normally, thus

o creating a toxic animal that is unnaturally obese and diseased.

o A conventional animal is fed an unnatural diet of chemicals and feed that it would never eat naturally. Conventional cows, for example, are fed ground up cow parts, pig parts, goat parts, and horse parts. Many of these ground-up animal parts are from diseased animals. Keep in mind that the cow is a vegetarian naturally and is not designed to be eating ground up animals diseased or otherwise.

o A conventional animal is slaughtered by being shot in the head with a bolt. The animal experiences pain and trauma. Adrenaline, which is poisonous, permeates the animal's tissue. The blood, which is loaded with toxins, also permeates the tissue. The trauma causes the energy field in and around the animal to become highly negative. The animal usually dies in its own urine and feces.

o A conventional animal is often aged, which means the animal flesh is hung in a dark room and allowed to rot. A green mold covers the rotting animal flesh. This green toxic mold is bacteria that tenderizes the meat, but it also fills the meat with more toxins.

o   An organic animal is given no drugs, so its meat is drug free.

o   An organic animal is allowed to roam naturally, grow at its normal rate, and is not diseased.

o   A grass-fed organic cow eats grass as it would in nature, and the grass has not been laced with chemical fertilizers, herbicides, and pesticides.

o   An organic animal that is also kosher is killed in the most humane way possible, by slicing its throat. The animal experiences no pain, is immediately drained of all blood, its internal organs are inspected to make sure the animal is healthy, and the tissue is salted to kill any bacteria.

o   Organic kosher meat is not aged.

When I learned all this, I decided to eat only kosher organic meat. For thirty days, every day, I ate some kosher organic meat. I tried to monitor whether I felt any difference. I couldn't detect anything specific or dramatic. I wasn't convinced that it was such a big deal. I decided to throw a barbecue and invited several friends over to my house. I went to the butcher and bought the best, highest quality steaks available, which happened to be conventional, Black Angus aged steaks. I cooked the steaks and served them to my guests. Each one raved about how delicious and tender the steaks were. Some said they were the best they'd ever eaten. I took one bite of mine and immediately felt odd. It was as if I was eating some "bad meat." Everyone else was enjoying theirs. I asked my friend to taste my steak. He loved it. So I took another bite. As I chewed and swallowed my forehead began to sweat, I got pale, and my stomach felt nauseated. I quickly excused myself, went to the bathroom and threw up. This happened because I had eaten only clean meat for so long my body immediately rejected the toxins. The bottom line is, chicken, duck, lamb, beef, and goat are all okay as long as they're organic and kosher. It may be a challenge to find kosher organic meats in some areas, but if you can it's worth it. If you *can't,* there are places online where you can order it and have it delivered via FedEx.

19. **Do not eat farm raised fish.**
Farm raised fish are given antibiotics and often treated with pesticides to combat sea lice. They're highly toxic, fattier than wild fish, and eating them can create inflammation in the body due to their higher ratio of Omega 6 to Omega 3s. A recent study in New York found that farm raised salmon was contaminated with PCBs. PCBs are toxins which have been implicated in causing a variety of diseases including cancer.

20. **Do not eat pork.**
Pork products are laced with disease and viruses. Nearly all pork in the U.S. comes from concentrated animal feeding operations or CAFOs. These toxic breeding grounds for pathogens are inhumane environments where the pigs are cramped on concrete and steel grates. Because there's so much bacteria in these horrible environments, the pigs are treated with large doses of antibiotics. Pigs digest whatever they eat quickly, within a few hours. Cows, for example, take up to twenty-four hours to digest their food. Because the pigs digest food quickly, more of the toxins remain in their system to be stored in their fatty tissues. We consume that tissue and it puts us at risk for illness. Another problem with pork is that pigs have virtually no sweat glands, so they don't release any toxins through perspiration like

other mammals. When you eat pork, you're eating all of the toxins the pig has.

21. **Do not eat shellfish.**

More people are allergic to shellfish than any other food. More people get sick from eating shellfish than any other food. More people die from eating shellfish than any other food. Any fish that does not have scales and fins should be avoided. This includes clams, mussels, shrimp, lobster, crab, squid, eel, catfish, shark, etc. The fish must have scales and fins. Catfish, for example, has fins but no scales. It is interesting that this is one of the kosher dietary laws. Today, we know that fish with scales and fins do not absorb the toxins in the water as readily as fish without both scales and fins. I grew up in the Boston area. I loved my shellfish more than any other seafood. Occasionally, a type of algae in the water called the "red tide" would infest the local shores. When this happened, warnings went out telling people not to eat any shellfish, because doing so could cause sickness or even death. However, you could eat the haddock, mackerel, or flounder. Fish that had scales and fins did not absorb the poisons into its edible flesh; however, shellfish or any fish that did not have both scales and fins would absorb the toxins and could kill you. Avoid all seafood that doesn't have scales and fins.

22. **If you can't eat it, don't put it on your skin.**

Whatever you put on the skin, which is our largest organ, gets absorbed and ends up in the body. Many of the products we put on our skin from antiperspirants, moisturizing lotions, cosmetics, insect repellents, sunscreens, and perfumes are so toxic that if you put them in your mouth they would poison you. I know for many of you it would be unrealistic to exclusively use products that were safe enough to eat. Remember, I said that if you can't do something 100 percent, do the best you can. You can eliminate many toxic products by replacing them with natural products. Extra virgin coconut oil (food grade, not the kind they sell in the drug store) is the best moisturizer you can use. It's emollient, antibacterial, and healthy for the skin. And it's sold in many grocery stores these days. It can also be used to remove makeup and cleanse the face and body. Spread it on and use a warm washcloth to wipe it off. Coconut oil can also be used to condition the hair. Put on before you shower and then wash out. Apple cider vinegar works as a toner for acne prone skin. It can also be used to cleanse the scalp and hair. If you can't eliminate all of the toxic products at least *reduce* the number of them that you put on your skin.

23. **Get an air purifier.**

I recommend an air purifier for your home, work space, and most importantly, your bedroom. Since you're breathing all night long, it would be a good idea to be breathing the cleanest, purest air you can. Your work space is the second most important. There are hundreds of types of air filters and air purifiers on the market. The best ones are so good they can even eliminate the black mold that's causing illness in many homes today. If you have an air purifier, use it regularly and change the filter as directed. If you don't have one, do some research and look for one that's highly rated and powerful enough to eliminate airborne mold.

24. **Use only nontoxic, organic cleaning supplies.**

Cleaning products used in the home have proven to be a leading cause of cancer in children. Toxic cleaning products suppress the immune system and cause disease. This occurs by inhaling the fumes, or through contact with the skin. Buy organic products or make your own with vinegar, baking soda, and lemon. White vinegar cleans glass, chrome, and tile. You can dilute it with water and you can add lemon juice if the smell bothers you. But when you clean with vinegar the smell goes away after a few minutes. Baking soda can clean ovens, sinks, and tubs. Baking soda *and* vinegar, together, create a powerful cleanser. Pour vinegar into a spray bottle; sprinkle baking soda onto a surface and spray it with the vinegar. It will bubble up and effectively clean and disinfect many surfaces in your home.

25. **Do not drink canned or bottled juice.**

All store-bought canned or bottled juice has been pasteurized making it toxic to the body. The filtering and processing used in juice manufacturing only increases and concentrates the amount of toxic chemicals. Drink only fresh juice made with organic ingredients.

26. **Avoid most sunscreens.**

They contain toxic chemicals. Oxybenzone, octinoxate and 4-MBC, which are in many sunscreens, are considered harmful and dangerous. Would you eat anything with names like that? If you can't eat it, don't put it on your skin. I don't believe in using *any* sunscreens, personally, but if you're at high risk for skin cancer or you live where the sun is particularly strong, it's understandable that you'd want some protection. My advice is to wear a hat and/or cover your body with light clothing in lieu of sunscreen. But if you absolutely need it, then at least look at the ingredients and avoid the poisons I noted.

27. **Take whole food supplements, rather than vitamins.**

There are many grades of individual vitamins. Unfortunately, most companies use the cheapest grades available. These inexpensive "vitamins" in many cases are chemically produced and are not natural. It's true that you are likely deficient in vitamins and minerals. The best way to correct this deficiency is by juicing. The second best way is to take *whole food supplements*. These are different from traditional, big-brand-name vitamin and mineral pills. Whole food supplements take organically produced vegetables and fruits and concentrate them into a convenient tablet. When you take a whole food supplement you're getting vitamins and minerals in a proportion that nature intended. You're also getting the enzymes and cofactors present in nature, which includes benefits that science hasn't even discovered yet.

28. **Do not use antiperspirants or deodorants.**
Antiperspirants and deodorants contain toxins, most notably aluminum. These poisons are being put on the skin close to the lymph nodes. Anything absorbed into the skin from the armpit gets drawn into the lymph system and travels to the breasts. I believe one of the major causes of breast cancer in women is the use of these poisonous products. A healthy person should not have an offensive odor if he or she bathes daily. The odor is caused by bacteria, and bathing should take care of that. If that's not enough, consider wiping your underarm with vinegar, preferably apple cider vinegar. Yes, you will smell it at first, but the vinegar odor will dissipate. Vinegar kills bacteria. You can also use baking soda, either like a powder, or wet it and make a thin paste. Some people use coconut oil, which also kills bacteria. Himalayan pink sea salt now comes in bars and can be used for bathing and deodorant. Remember, if you can't eat it, don't put it on your skin. If you *must* use deodorant, look for all natural products that don't contain chemicals.

29. **Do not eat processed flour.**
White processed flour is similar to white sugar in that consuming it raises the blood sugar level. Processed flour comes

from grain that's been chemically treated in the growing process. It's also stripped of its natural fiber and nutrients, and chemically bleached to make it white. White flour mixed with water makes paste. You use it to make papi-er-mâché. It turns hard as a rock. And that's what happens when you eat it. It is an unnatural product that the body has difficulty digesting. It has little nutritional value, no life energy, spikes your insulin, and causes constipation. Avoid breads, cakes, cookies, pasta and anything else made with white flour. I don't recommend whole wheat flour either, because the wheat supply has been modified and it's no longer a natural product. In place of breads and pasta, eat real grains: oatmeal, brown rice, and quinoa.

30. **Eat nothing that says "fat-free" on the label.**

    Food companies want you to buy their products. Whatever the hot button is at the time will determine what their marketing people decide goes on the label. "Fat free" does not mean "healthy." Most fat free products mask the loss of taste (due to removing the fat) by loading them with sugar and chemicals. These things are toxic and detrimental to your health.

31. **Eat nothing that says "sugar-free" on the label.**

    If it says sugar free on the label there's a good chance the product is laced with artificial sweeteners. Don't buy it. Obviously, there are many foods that naturally don't contain sugar and I'm not talking about those. I'm talking about processed snacks in the grocery. Avoid them. They're not going to help you lose weight. Eating real, unprocessed food will help you lose weight.

32. **Eat nothing that says "low carbs" or "net carbs" on the label.**

    The term "net carbs" is a big scam. Manufacturers load these products with chemicals and artificial sweeteners that they claim have negligible results on insulin levels, so they don't count these real carbohydrates in the net carb number. It's nonsense. A product that says it has two net carbs could have as many as forty grams of real carbohydrates. Do not buy these products, as you know that the manufacturers are simply trying to take advantage of a fad to sell you their products. Learn about glycemic index and try to eat foods with a lower glycemic index. You don't need to count carbs. If you're not eating processed flour, and instead eating whole grains, and if you're eliminating sugar and processed foods, you don't need to worry about "net carbs."

33. **Do not eat "food bars."**

Food bars are man-made products that are filled with chemicals to provide good taste. They're highly processed and should be avoided. There *are* a few all-raw, organic food bars and these are okay. Be sure to read the ingredient list.

34. **Do not eat diet or protein shakes.**

Like food bars, these are produced by companies whose goal is to make them taste great using the cheapest ingredients possible. They often have chemical additives and/or sugar. Make your own shakes at home with a blender using real ingredients. Smoothies are a great way to get your fruits and vegetables. You can use nuts, nut butters, and seeds to increase the protein content. Chia seeds are a good source of protein and blend well.

35. **Stay away from hot tubs, steam rooms, and chlorine swimming pools.**

Swimming pools and hot tubs are filled with water that's loaded with chlorine. Chlorine is a poisonous chemical. People think swimming in a pool, or relaxing in a hot tub is healthy. The exact opposite is true. They suppress your immune system, dry your skin, and load your body with high levels of chlorine, which can scar your arteries and lead to heart disease. The steam pouring into the steam room is from regular tap water that's loaded with contaminants. A steam room is, in fact, a poisonous gas chamber. Swimming is excellent in the ocean or in a lake. If you have a pool or hot tub, inquire about a filtration system where no chlorine or chemicals are used. The system I use employs ozone and oxygen to purify the water. No chlorine or chemicals are put into my pool or hot tub. If you can't drink the water, don't swim in it. Some people may say you can't drink lake water or ocean water, and that's true. But those waters are living, vitalized natural waters. Chlorinated swimming pools are something not found in nature.

36. Don't use air fresheners.

Don't spray anything in the air. Avoid solid air fresheners and the plug-in variety. All they do is put toxic chemicals in the air. It's insane. In my bathrooms I do have a can of organic citrus oil, which is nontoxic and can be purchased at most health food stores. Read the labels. Use 100 percent organic essential oils or air purification systems (filters) to eliminate offensive odors.

37. Eliminate fluorescent lighting.

Fluorescent lighting is irritating to the body. It makes you tired and weakens the immune system. Get rid of all florescent lighting and replace it with full spectrum lighting. Full spectrum lighting is similar to natural sunlight, and can have health benefits, most notably increased energy and alleviation of depression.

38. Reduce air conditioning.

Generally, air conditioning is not healthy. It makes the air unnatural. And poorly maintained units can contribute to airborne bacteria and fungi. In some climates, it's impossible to live without air conditioning. I get that. But use it less and you'll see a decrease in the amount of colds and flu you get. Where possible, use ceiling fans instead.

39. **Avoid dry cleaning.**

The chemicals in dry cleaning are toxic poisons. Allowing them to come in contact with your skin increases risk of disease. The chemicals have been linked to cancer, liver and nervous system damage, infertility, and hormonal disturbances. Hand wash delicate clothes when possible, or have them laundered and pressed rather than dry cleaned. For garments where that's not feasible, look for dry cleaners that specify that they do not use toxic chemicals.

40. **Buy a vacuum cleaner with a HEPA filter.**

Using a vacuum with a HEPA filter will help reduce the toxins in your home. When you walk into your house from the outside, you track inside environmental toxins and all kinds of allergens. Using a vacuum with a good filter can help people with asthma and allergies. The filter traps fine particles, which benefits everyone, even non-allergy sufferers.

Implementing the recommendations above will reduce the number of toxins going into your body and can also cure disease. These are in fact "natural cures." I've seen people with diabetes stop eating in fast food restaurants and in three weeks they no longer had diabetes. I've seen people who suffer from migraine headaches and constipation problems stop eating pasteurized and homogenized dairy products and the migraines stopped and they became regular. I've seen people with horrible skin rashes and acne use a shower filter and find that their symptoms disappeared, their skin become smooth and beautiful again. Don't be misled into thinking that things as simple as these are not cures. These things are causing your illnesses, and eliminating them can cure you.

C. You must address your nutritional deficiencies.

Many, if not all, diseases are caused at least in part by nutritional deficiencies.

By now, hopefully you understand that you have nutritional deficiencies and you also understand *why* you have them. The reason you're deficient in nutrients is because the food is grown and processed in such a way that its nutritional value is stripped from it before it even reaches you. And because we have so many toxins in our body, we have difficulty absorbing what little nutrition we *are* getting from our food. Many, if not all, diseases are caused at least in part by nutritional deficiencies. If you want to prevent and cure disease you must mitigate your nutritional deficiencies. So let me give you a list of dos and don'ts designed to help your body retain nutrients. For many of you this will be the miraculous all natural cure that you've been looking for.

1. **Eat more fresh organic fruits and vegetables.**
   You don't have to be a vegetarian to be healthy. However, the healthiest people eat a lot of fresh, organic fruits and vegetables. If you were to do just one thing to improve your level of nutrition, I would tell you to eat four pieces of fresh fruit per day and two big raw salads full of vegetables. If you changed nothing else in your diet and just added those two things, many medical conditions would disappear.

2. **Buy a juice machine and use it.**
   Our current food supply is dramatically depleted of vital vitamins and minerals. Organic produce has up to ten times more vitamins and minerals than nonorganic, and it has none of the poisonous residues from the chemical fertilizers, pesticides, and fungicides. Even so, because the soil is

so depleted, organic produce still has less nutritional value than the same produce had fifty years ago. Therefore, it's difficult to get enough of the necessary vitamins, minerals, and enzymes just by eating food. And remember, because of all of the toxins you've ingested, your ability to absorb these nutrients is reduced. Even if you ate nothing but raw, uncooked organic fruits, vegetables, nuts, and seeds, your body would still have nutritional deficiencies. The best way to correct this is to make fresh juice using organic fruits and vegetables. Drinking three to four glasses of fresh juice gives your body a good dose of living enzymes, as well as many vitamins and minerals in their natural state as nature intended.

3. **Eat raw organic nuts and seeds.**

    Raw means uncooked. Stay away from roasted and salted nuts and seeds. Ideally, buy them in the shell; they retain more nutrients. There's tremendous life force in nuts and seeds. They're great to snack on throughout the day. One caveat: They're dense in calories and high in fat. So try to keep your snacking to between one to three ounces a day.

4. **Get natural sunlight.**

    Go for a walk in the sun. Your body benefits from sunlight. Do not use sunglasses. The sun enters through the eyes and stimulates energy in the entire body. Let some of your skin be exposed to the sun, because sunlight on the skin helps the body produce much needed Vitamin D. This natural source of Vitamin D dramatically reduces the risk of developing several kinds of cancer. Remember, it's the sun that creates growth in plants. The solar energy from sun can be alkalizing to the body; it reduces depression and strengthens the immune system.

5. **Eat an organic apple a day.**

   It's true, an apple a day keeps the doctor away! This is a "natural cure" for dozens of diseases. It is in fact a superfood.

6. **Take all natural Vitamin E.**

   One of the most important vitamins you are deficient in, in my opinion, is Vitamin E. Taking Vitamin E can prevent a number of conditions including heart disease as well as eliminate varicose veins, improve sexual performance, reduce or alleviate depression,and a whole host of other disorders.

7. **Take liquid colloidal minerals daily.**

   You are deficient in minerals. Nutritional deficiencies lead to disease. Correcting these deficiencies cures disease. Colloidal minerals provide structure to tissues in your body. They also support an adequate acid-base balance in your body. They support the many processes of enzymes as well.

8. **Drink the "magic juices."**

   There are several fruits that have miraculous healing properties in the body. These are: noni, goji, mangosteen, acai berry and aloe vera. Aloe vera is technically a succulent plant, but I'm including it in this group. Some of these fruits are from other parts of the world and so they're difficult to buy fresh. While I generally discourage one from buying bottled juice, most of these must be purchased bottled. Unfortunately, they're pasteurized, because the government requires that. Pasteurization is not ideal, however the positive outweighs the negative in this case. I highly encourage you to buy and drink these juices. They provide super nutrition and they help cleanse and detoxify the body as well.

9. **Take a whole food supplement daily.**

   Whole food supplements are not synthetic vitamins and minerals. They are "concentrated real food." They contain nutrients, living enzymes, and life force energy in the proportion that nature intended. Whole food supplements include chlorella, blue-green algae, spirulina, royal jelly, and other types of concentrated whole herbs, plants, dehydrated juices, and/or sprouts. Remember, your body is deficient in vitamins, minerals and enzymes. There's no way you can get all of the nutrients you need just by eating food. You would have to eat ten to twenty times the amount of food you're eating now, and it would all have to be organic for you to meet your minimum nutritional needs. Since nutritional deficiencies cause disease, it's essential that you take a supplement with the proper amount of vitamins, minerals, and enzymes to help your body to operate at its best, and prevent diseases from developing.

10. **Eat raw organic honey, bee propolis, royal jelly, and bee pollen.**

Raw organic bee products and honey are super nutritious foods. Royal jelly, for example, is an excellent health tonic that has been found to reduce tumors. It benefits the immune system and improves a number of conditions including asthma, allergies, insomnia, and high cholesterol. It also helps combat menopausal symptoms, stomach ulcers, liver disease, pancreatitis, kidney disease and bone fractures. Bee pollen boosts the immune system, treats allergies and can prevent the onset of asthma. It also aids digestion. Take bee products with meals for the best absorption.

11. **Get an oxygen water cooler.**

For a variety of reasons, your body is deficient in oxygen. Bringing the level of oxygen to where it should be alkalizes the body and creates an environment where disease cannot exist. One of the best ways to get more oxygen into the body is through water. Do not buy oxygenated water at the store. The oxygen dissipates rapidly and by the time you buy it, any oxygen that was added is likely gone. I have water coolers in my home and office that add the oxygen when the water is dispensed. Most people feel an immediate rush of energy and increased vitality.

12. **Take digestive enzymes.**

One of the main causes of indigestion, heartburn, gas, bloating, and constipation is a lack of digestive enzymes in the stomach and intestine. Because of antibiotics, other prescription and nonprescription drugs, chlorinated and fluoridated water, most people don't have enough digestive enzymes in their system, which slows the metabolism and blocks the absorption of nutrients. It's essential to take digestive enzymes for a period of time until your body is cleansed and rejuvenated, and can produce the correct amount on its own. Taking digestive enzymes can eliminate acid reflux, heartburn, indigestion, gas, bloating, and constipation. The majority of people who begin taking digestive enzymes lose between five and ten pounds in the first thirty days.

13. **Eat probiotic foods.**

Probiotic foods contain microorganisms that are similar to the microorganisms found in the human digestive system. They benefit the immune system. Organic yogurt with live cultures is a good source of probiotics. Fermented foods like miso, sauerkraut, tempeh, and kimchi are also good sources.

14. **Use Himalayan pink sea salt.**

Regular table salt is poison. Sea salt is infinitely better for you. Himalayan pink sea salt contains the full spectrum of minerals and trace elements. Replacing your white nutrient stripped salt with Himalayan pink sea salt will help balance your body's pH and also improve circulation. Regular table salt is considered unhealthy and can exacerbate high blood pressure. This sea salt, used in moderation (too much of *any* form of sodium is not good), can help normalize blood pressure.

15. **Eat organic dark chocolate.**

Dark chocolate has a lot of antioxidants. Antioxidants help rid the body of free radicals that cause oxidative damage to the cells. This slows the aging process, and also protects against some forms of cancer. Dark chocolate benefits the heart by lowering blood pressure. It benefits the brain by increasing blood flow, which helps cognitive function. Don't over indulge, because it's also high in fat and calories, but an ounce a day will benefit your health without weight gain. Be sure that the kind of dark chocolate you're eating is 70 percent cacao, or higher to receive the benefits.

16. **Take an omega-3 supplement.**

Omega-3s (essential fatty acids) help lower triglycerides and blood pressure. They also help treat arthritis and depression. They're primarily available in fish oil capsules, (purchase a brand that assures *no mercury*), but they're also available as flaxseed oil capsules. They reduce inflammation throughout the body, which assists in disease prevention.

17. **Eat snacks.**

Don't go hungry. What I mean by *eat snacks* is eat in between meals if you're hungry. However, my definition of snack and your definition of snack are probably two different things. My definition of "snack" is: organic apples, pears, or other organic fruit, organic raw nuts and seeds, organic raw celery, carrots, cucumbers or other vegetables, or freshly made juices, organic chicken salad, tuna salad, or other organic beef or poultry... you get the idea. I mean healthy snacks, not junk food or sweets. And my point is, you don't need to go hungry to be healthy.

As I've said repeatedly, you are nutritionally deficient. Virtually *every* disease has been linked to nutritional deficiencies and research is conclusive that when nutritional deficiencies are addressed many diseases vanish. Adding appropriate snacks is one way to bolster your level of nutrition. Food is medicine. So be sure that you're eating the healthiest foods possible. Can eating some raw organic honey cure a disease? Can eating an organic apple cure a disease? Can drinking some goji juice or mangosteen juice cure a disease? The answer: Absolutely. You bet it can.

D. Neutralize electromagnetic chaos

As you now know, electromagnetic chaos can cause your body to develop disease. We can't eliminate electromagnetic chaos, but we can reduce our exposure to it. Reducing, eliminating, or neutralizing these powerful negative frequencies can and does result in the "curing" of symptoms and disease. I've seen men with erectile dysfunction and prostate cancer cured by simply discontinuing the use of laptop computers. Why? Because in their case the powerful wireless devices in the laptops were causing their disease. I've seen people with migraines, fatigue, and depression be cured just by wearing an electromagnetic chaos eliminator because their symptoms were caused by sitting in front of a computer screen all day long at work. Cell phones do cause cancer. Laptop computers do cause cancer. High-definition TVs do cause cancer. As a matter of fact, all of these things not only cause cancer, but they also suppress the body's immune system and make us susceptible to all kinds of diseases. The manufacturers of these devices deny these allegations, of course, because there's too much money to be lost. Remember, it's always all about the money. But there are scientists and researchers who assert that these devices cause disease. So let me give you some recommendations for managing electromagnetic chaos.

1. **Use crystals to neutralize electromagnetic chaos.**

   As I mentioned, we're being bombarded by electromagnetic energy from hundreds of sources, including satellites, high-tension power lines, computers, cell phones, global positioning systems in our cars, wireless telephones, remote controls, high-definition TVs, etc. We can't eliminate the electromagnetic energy around us. We can only do things to neutralize the negative effects. Crystals help neutralize these negative energies. Some can be put in your home or office near your computer and minimize the negative energy in the space around you; others can be carried in your purse or pocket, or worn as a pendant. When I say *crystals*, I'm speaking of naturally formed crystals of quartz, amethyst, etc., not the kind on a chandelier. You can find them online and also in stores that specialize in gem stones and new age material. They are inexpensive and work brilliantly.

2. **Use electronic and wireless devices less.**

   It appears that some of the most negative effects of electromagnetic energy come from wireless devices such as cell phones, laptops, as well as high-definition TVs. I know it's impossible to eliminate the use of these devices; however, you should at least be aware of their powerful adverse effects and limit their use as best as you can.

3. **Reduce TV time.**

   Televisions produce unhealthy electromagnetic energy. High-definition televisions have an *especially* powerful negative electromagnetic energy. The images on TV are largely stress invoking. This doesn't mean you can never watch it, but if you're watching TV every night, seven days a week and you're watching things that are violent or otherwise stressful, that's not conducive to healing or maintaining good health.

4. **Get a magnetic mattress pad.**

   The Earth, at one time, had a magnetic level (called gauss) of 4.0. Today the Earth's gauss is .04. Sleeping on a mattress pad filled with magnets stimulates energy flowing through the body as nature intended. It has been said to alleviate pain, slow the aging process, increase energy, and help alkalize the body.

5. **Use magnetic finger and toe rings.**

   These are inexpensive and easy to use. Simply wear a specially designed magnetic ring on the small finger of each hand, and if you want even more benefit, wear the toe brace on each foot. These are worn while you sleep. The health benefits seem to be almost unbelievable. This device appears to radically slow the aging process. People report looking and feeling younger as time goes on.

6. **Stay away from electric tumble dryers.**

   These devices produce massive amounts of positive ions. Positive ions suppress the immune system, make you fatigued, and can cause depression and anxiety. Do this experiment: Go to a Laundromat and sit in front of the tumble dryers in operation, and notice how you feel after just thirty minutes. Then notice how you feel for the rest of the day. Compare this to taking a walk on the beach or being near running water, or an area with lots of trees. These conditions produce life-enhancing negative ions. The comparison in how you feel can be dramatic. The clothes that come out of the tumble dryer are also charged with these ions that have a negative effect on your emotions and physiology. You will actually feel better if you wear clothes that have been line dried in fresh air.

7. **Add living plants to your home.**

   Real living plants add oxygen to the air, balance the energy in the space, produce life-enhancing negative ions, and are incredibly beneficial to the health of human beings. Fill your house with living plants and flowers. You will feel the difference and benefit from the moment you do it.

8. **Wear white.**

   Colors affect energy. The closer you get to white, the more positive energy you bring into your energetic field. This may not be practical in everyday situations; however, having some white or light colored clothing as your general around-the-house attire can make you feel much better.

9. **Use feng shui in your home and office.**

   This ancient method of arranging things allows energy to flow better, reducing stress, increasing prosperity, and generating vibrant health.

As simple as some of these things seem, they *can* be the "natural cure" you're looking for. I know there are a lot of recommendations and it's unlikely that you'll do every single one. Do as many as you can. With the majority of people one thing is not the cause of their illnesses, it's a combination of things. And often one thing is not going to be the cure. You need to do a variety of things to change your health. You must change your lifestyle. If you're not well, the lifestyle you were experiencing (the way you took care of yourself) created the conditions for sickness to develop. So adopt a number of these positive changes to improve the quality of your lifestyle and the quality of your health will improve as well.

E. You must reduce stress.

Stress is the silent killer. Mental and emotional stress affects every cell in the body. The mind can turn the body's pH from acidic to alkaline in a matter of minutes. Stress can adversely affect your body's genetic makeup. The mind can positively or negatively affect DNA. If you want to prevent disease, be happy, eliminate depression and fatigue, and cure illness, you must reduce stress in your body. It is impossible to "eliminate *all* stress," but you can certainly *reduce* stress. Can eliminating stress cure a disease? The surprising answer is *yes*. Healthcare practitioners around the world have proven repeatedly that by simply reducing stress, diseases are cured. The "placebo affect" has shown that up to 40 percent of people cure themselves with nothing more than their thoughts. That comes directly from the pharmaceutical industry's own literature and it's *a natural cure they don't want you to know about.*

> Stress can adversely affect your body's genetic makeup

So let me give you a list of what *I* think are the most powerful ways to reduce stress. I recommend doing as many of these things as you can. And I urge you to begin doing them as soon and as often as you can.

1. **Listen to de-stressing CDs.**

    One of the best ways to eliminate stress is to regularly listen to CDs specifically designed for that purpose. You can find them online. You need headphones when you use this specially created music (and in some cases words) because the frequencies are designed in such a way that they go into one ear or the other and at carefully selected time intervals. These CDs stimulate the brain to release healing hormones, and dramatically release tension that's been trapped in the body. Your pH levels can be radically changed in a matter of minutes with these powerful tools.

2. **Meditate.**

   There are many forms of meditation to choose from. You can practice the technique you prefer if you have one. Or if you're new to meditation, start by taking some time, perhaps once a day, to sit in silence for several minutes. Start off with 15 minutes and try to build up to 30 minutes or even an hour if you can. Close your eyes and be still. Sit or lie in a comfortable position and do nothing but focus on your breath. As thoughts come up, let them go and bring your attention back to your breath. If you prefer, you can focus on a word like "peace," but try to quiet your mind and allow yourself to be still in silence. Doing this regularly has healing benefits. It's good for the brain, and over time, it can improve your overall health and wellbeing.

3. **Laugh.**

   Laughing is one of the most powerfully beneficial and healing things you can do. Children laugh, on average, 10,000 times per week. Adults laugh, on average, five times per week. Laughing stimulates the immune system, reduces depression and alkalizes the body. In the book *The Anatomy of an Illness*, we hear the amazing story of a cancer patient who, given six months to live, used laughter to eliminate his cancer. The popular documentary *The Secret* showed a woman who watched funny movies and laughed each day to eradicate her breast cancer quickly and without radiation or chemotherapy. Laugh daily, as often as you can, even if you have nothing to laugh about. You'll feel better and your body will be healthier.

4. **Smile.**

   The physical act of smiling strengthens the immune system and releases endorphins from the brain, making you feel better. The act of smiling also changes your energetic field, as evidenced by Kirlian photography. Make it a habit to notice if you're smiling or not. Smile for no reason and do it often.

5. **Get and give hugs.**

Human contact is essential in order to thrive. Babies who are given all of the nutrition they need, but receive no physical contact grow less, cry more, and come down with more illnesses than babies who are cuddled regularly. Our immune systems are strengthened when we physically hug another human being. Ask yourself how many hugs you gave and got yesterday. You should be hugging every day as often as possible. It's a gratifying way to experience increased health.

6. **Speak powerful words.**

Words create. What you say is what you get. Most people get hung by their own tongue. When you say something you energetically put the wheels in motion that will manifest it into reality. Speak positively and use words as a tool to make what you desire come to pass. Say things like: I am healthy, I am happy, I am excited about life. Or say whatever is it that you want to occur. Say it as if it's true, and in the present tense, not: I *want* to be healthy. Instead affirm: I *am* healthy. It doesn't matter if you are not actually healthy in the moment. You are using the right words to make it so. Speaking in these affirmative ways impresses your subconscious mind powerfully. If you say I *want* something, rather than I *am* or I *have*, your subconscious will obediently agree with what you say and you will remain *wanting* that thing.

7. **Don't use a cell phone and drive at the same time.**

Holding a cell phone and driving is illegal in many states, as it should be, since it selfishly endangers others. But I discourage hands-free cell phone use as well. Driving is stressful enough. When you're talking on a cell phone and driving simultaneously, the physical and psychological stress can be even greater. If you're trying to reduce stress in order to bring your body into balance, driving and talking on the phone is not going to help. When driving, consider listening to soothing music to help counter the stress. Just make sure it's not so soothing that it puts you to sleep.

8. **Sleep eight hours.**

Ideally, get a full eight hours of solid, deep, restful sleep every night. This is easier said than done, but do what you can to get there. Power down your electronics at least an hour before bed. Don't have them on in your bedroom, especially if they emit any light. Even a small amount of light can affect sleep quality. Use earplugs if noise keeps you awake. If your mattress isn't comfortable replace it. Set the temperature where it's not too hot or too cold. Use comfortable sleepwear. Avoid caffeine within several hours of going to bed and avoid eating too close to bedtime. If drinking causes you to go to the bathroom several times a night, consider drinking your fluids earlier in the day and stop ingesting them a couple of hours before bed so you can sleep through the night.

9. **Rest from Friday sundown to Saturday sundown.**

Each week the moon cycles are in position to promote healing and rejuvenation in the body. Resting during this time promotes the optimal rejuvenation of your cells. "Rest" doesn't mean lying in your bed, necessarily, but if you're that tired, it's fine. Rest means no work, or stressful obligations. Have family time, or consider silent time with yourself to read, write in a journal, think your own thoughts, plan your next week... Whatever, just so long as you give your body some time to wind down. You can't be your best if you never take the time to replenish your energy. Scheduling the time to do that can really help you find balance in your life.

10. **Go to bed at approximately 10:00 p.m. and arise at approximately 6:00 a.m.**

In Ayurvedic medicine it is believed that there are cycles that are the most conducive for certain activities. Going to bed at 10:00 p.m. and rising at 6:00 a.m. appears to allow the body to rest the deepest, rejuvenate the most, and gives one the most energy throughout the day. Hormones that heal the body are released only between 10:00 p.m. and 2:00 a.m., and they're only released when the body is in deep sleep.

11. **Take an afternoon fifteen minute break.**

Most people wake up to an alarm, rush to work, stress, worry and work all day, rush to get home, eat a meal, and sit in front of the television. Then they go to bed and prepare to repeat the process again the next day. A fifteen minute relaxation break, ideally using special music or relaxation CDs, allows the body a mini-rest to decompress, and rejuvenate sufficiently to get you through the rest of the day with better energy and clarity.

12. **Get rolfing.**

Rolfing is a type of deep-tissue massage technique that releases the fasciae (connective tissues between the muscle and the bone) and dramatically improves posture and balance, and integrates the entire body. Rolfing is generally done once per week for fifteen weeks. Each session is like a deep-tissue massage and takes approximately an hour and a half. You can find trained Rolfing practitioners in your area. I highly recommend this.

13. **Don't read the newspaper.**

Most of us get our news online so this applies to online reading as well. You can't bombard your mind with negative thoughts and expect your body's pH to remain alkaline. The newspaper is filled with negativity, which causes anxiety. The news is almost always misleading, slanted, or in some cases, completely untrue. So more often than not, it's not the best use of your energy to focus on it. Yes, we live in the real world and we want to know what's going on, but it's problematic to dwell on and react to a negative story. The emotions become involved and stress levels go up. When you feel yourself getting anxious, realize that your pH is becoming more acidic. Our goal is to keep your pH level alkaline.

14. **Avoid watching the news.**

Watching the news on television fills your mind with negative images that can have a profound effect on wellbeing. I've done my own study and found that one's pH level can go from a healthy alkaline state, to the cancer-prone acidic state after just thirty minutes of watching a stressful news broadcast. If you want to stay up on current events glance at the major headlines, or briefly listen to the radio news and then move on with your day. If there's something you *really* need to know, someone will surely tell you. Don't dwell on stressful stories when you're trying to heal yourself, or stay well.

15. **Have sex regularly.**

There are many benefits to sexual activity, including strengthening the immune system, reducing stress, lowering blood pressure, and improving sleep quality. There have even been studies suggesting that having sex a few times a week can make both men and women look several years younger. This study also said that the benefits came with having sex with a consistent partner. (I'm not telling you to go out and have a bunch of one night stands.) Casual sex would actually be detrimental and not lead to stress reduction.

16. **Commit reckless acts of kindness.**

Each day make it a goal, then ultimately a habit to be kind to everyone you meet. The act of showing kindness stimulates the body's immune system and gives one a greater sense of peace. It causes stress when you interact with hostility or mean-spiritedness toward another. If you're annoyed, in the moment, you may think you feel better by snapping at someone or being rude, but the body says otherwise by becoming stressed. (Remember those pH levels?) We're all connected and what goes around comes around. So send out kindness and you can relax, knowing that that's what you have coming back to you.

17. **Listen to nice music.**

   Certain kinds of music have been shown to kill plants and to suppress the immune system in humans. Certain music also has been shown to make the body acidic. Baroque classical music seems to promote health and vitality in plants, and it seems to encourage the same in humans. You can sense which types of music are healing and relaxing for you. It's different for everyone, but the point is to recognize what makes you feel good and peaceful, rather than anxious, because the music that puts you at ease is going to benefit your health.

18. **Get out of debt.**

   Financial pressure causes an increase in stress, which can lead to disease. There are several organizations that can assist you in managing, reducing, and eliminating debt. Consider Debtors Anonymous if you think you have a chronic problem. When you free yourself from financial worry you're more likely to be relaxed, happier and healthier.

19. **Drive less.**

   Driving causes a lot of stress. If you're driving a lot in your life, see if you can make any changes. Car pool? Public transportation? Even making a switch a couple of times a week can make a difference if you commute regularly. If you take a bus or train, you can rest on the way, or catch up on reading so you don't have to be in constant stress mode the entire trip. If you live in a city, but you drive everywhere, consider walking, riding a bike, or taking a bus now and then for a break from driving. It'll be better for you *and* for the environment.

20. **Be thankful.**

Thoughts are things. Thoughts are powerful. When you wake up in the morning, take a moment to be thankful for the day. Before you eat a meal, take a moment and be thankful for the food. Before you go to bed, reflect and be thankful for the people and experiences you have. Living a life of gratitude creates happiness and peace, reduces stress, and promotes general health.

21. **Get an inversion table.**

Machines are available online and in fitness equipment stores that allow you to tilt your body into an inverted position or hang completely upside down. This process is believed to decompress the spine, relieve back pain, increase blood and oxygen to the brain, reduce stress and potentially slow the aging process. I own one of these machines myself and use it a few times a week. It only takes three minutes and you feel absolutely fantastic.

22. **Use foot orthotics.**

Good foot orthotics can promote general health and can eliminate foot, joint, and back pain. If you walk a lot, have an injury that makes walking painful, or you have arthritis or diabetes, this is worth looking into. Some prescribers/sellers are better than others. Be sure to work with a company or doctor who specializes in orthotics and get recommendations.

23. **Get a range of motion machine.**

How would you like to get the benefits of thirty minutes of aerobics, forty-five minutes of stretching, and forty-five minutes of strength training in just four minutes? There's a machine called the "range of motion machine" which does just that. It's expensive, but highly recommended.

24. **Be lighthearted.**

There are tens of thousands of people around the world who live past the age of one hundred. Research conducted on these centenarians has found that one of the major common denominators is that they take life lightly. They strive to be happy. It's a good reminder. Hold grudges less. Smile more. Don't stress over things unnecessarily. Remember, stress is one of the things that contribute to an acidic pH, which creates an environment conducive to disease.

25. **Stay away from psychiatrists.**

Psychiatrists almost always prescribe drugs to their patients. These drugs are some of the most dangerous pharmaceuticals available today. Did you know that many of the violent acts committed in schools in the past several years were perpetrated by someone who had either taken, or was currently taking a psychiatric drug? The research has become so compelling that there are warnings that certain psychiatric drugs actually increase the propensity to commit suicide. Avoid psychiatrists and the drugs they prescribe.

26. **Do not use an alarm clock.**

Or if you do, don't use one that shocks you awake with a loud, harsh noise. Most people wake to the sound of a loud alarm clock. This shocks the system and starts the body off in a stress mode for the day. It's important, and better for you, to awaken slowly and gently. There are alarm clocks that wake you with gentle tones or natural sounds like ocean waves that start off low in volume and slowly get louder. There are also clocks that wake you with a light that gradually increases in brightness. This little change in the way you awaken can have profound effects on your emotions and your body's pH.

27. **Use aromatherapy.**

Smells have a powerful effect on the body. Certain smells evoke chemical reactions. They can be soothing and healing. Essential oils have many health benefits in addition to wonderfully pleasant aromas. Seek out an aromatherapy expert to help you choose the essential oils and aromas specifically for you.

28. **Use Thought Field Therapy or the Emotional Freedom Technique (tapping).**

Phobias, stress, compulsions, and other dysfunctional problems can be treated by using a technique that involves tapping meridian points on the body with one's fingers. Thought Field Therapy was developed by Roger Callahan. His book is called *Tapping the Power Within*. The Emotional Freedom Technique, developed by Gary Craig, is a similar modality. Both approaches are derived from acupuncture and help a person release energy blockages.

29. **Get a pet.**

Research indicates that having a pet leads to a longer life and less disease. Pets give unconditional love and allow us a nonjudgmental being to give love to. The process of being loved and giving love strengthens our immune system, reduces stress, and has a variety of emotional and physical benefits.

30. **Write down goals.**

Write down what you want. Something magical occurs when you physically write down the things you want in life. This is one of the most powerful secrets used by the super wealthy. Just as I advised you how to speak your powerful thoughts earlier (*I am* healthy, rather than *I want to be* healthy), write powerful words. You might even write then with gratitude as if they're already true. For example: "Thank you for my healing," as if it's already accomplished.

31. **Plant a garden.**

    Being in the physical universe, working with living things and creating things with our hands is incredibly beneficial. Working in a garden provides an outdoor environment, exercise, stress reduction, and many more mental, emotional, and physical benefits. It's awe-inspiring to start with a tiny seed or a small plant and watch it flourish into something amazing. Gardening will connect you with how wonderful and creative the universe is.

32. **Cook.**

    When we create something with our hands we benefit emotionally and physically. When you cook food from scratch you take a much needed mental break, and you can create great tasting, incredibly healthy meals. I personally cook almost every day.

33. **Don't eat late.**

    It is best to stop eating at 7:00 p.m. You'll sleep better, wake more refreshed, and find it easier to manage your weight.

34. **Dance and sing.**

    Dancing and singing are great ways to release stress in the body. They are fun, and have a positive impact on our emotions and our physiology. Sing in the shower, or the car, if you're shy. Dance while you brush your teeth. However you do it, let dancing and singing be an expression of the joy within you. The more you express joy, the more you'll create within your life.

35. **Find your life's purpose.**

I put this last, although it's the most important. The reason it's last is because it is probably the hardest. Most people go throughout life without ever finding their true life's purpose. I can tell you from experience how stressful life can be when you are going day after day feeling like you're not doing what you were put on Earth to do. I experienced that myself early in my career when my focus was solely on making money at all costs. Today, my stress levels are at the lowest they've ever been, yet the amount of stressors in my life are the highest. Why? Because I've found my life's purpose, and that is to expose corporate and government corruption, and help people cure themselves of disease without drugs and surgery. My life is no longer about making money. Instead, I'm motivated to get true, honest healing information to people around the world, and to stop the insatiable greed going on primarily in the pharmaceutical companies and healthcare industry all around the globe.

Finding your life purpose, I believe, can help you be happier and healthier than ever before. It is hard to do, but I encourage you to consider where you are, and what your purpose is. Maybe your purpose is to help others achieve their purpose. Maybe your purpose in life is to make your own home and family happy and healthy. Maybe it's to help support me in my quest of educating people around the world on natural healing methods. I gratefully ask that you support me by reading the monthly newsletter (which can be ordered at www.NaturalCuresBook.com/newsletter) and writing me with your success stories at mystory@NaturalCuresSuccess. com. Stay connected so you can keep up with new articles. They'll be helpful to you in many areas of your life. I'd also love for you to direct positive energy and thoughts toward me and my mission. I am thanking you in advance for your support, and I hope the information in this book will be the miracle you've been looking for.

There you have my basic list of things to do and things to avoid that can bring your body back to a state of balance, eliminating disease and illness. It would be silly for anyone to believe that a person could do *all* of these things *all of the time*. Ideally, do as many as you can as often as you can. Doing even a little bit is better than none at all. For example, you may not be able to eliminate something 100 percent. At least cut back or reduce, or try eliminating it for a day or two. The more you do these things, and the more often you do them, the healthier and younger you will feel.

What you have in this chapter is what I believe to be the method to cure the incurable; the secrets to a long healthy disease-free life, full of energy and vitality, and in my opinion, the fountain of youth. These are some of the cures *they don't want you to know about.* Since I strongly believe that the cause of all disease is too many toxins in the body, nutritional deficiencies, exposure to electromagnetic chaos, and stress, the way to prevent and cure every disease is simply eliminate toxins in the body, eliminate nutritional deficiencies, eliminate or reduce exposure to electromagnetic chaos, and eliminate or reduce stress. The suggestions are simple, yet powerful and effective. I encourage you to start implementing some of these things immediately. I believe that you'll start feeling better remarkably quickly. I get letters and emails every week with people telling me of their success as they've been implementing the recommendations

> These techniques are powerful because they address the "cause" of all disease and illness.

in this chapter. These techniques are powerful because they address the "cause" of all disease and illness.

Now, I want to specifically address a very important issue facing not only America, but people all over the world. That issue is... LOSING WEIGHT! Let's learn the truth about why you're fat and how to lose weight once and for all, and keep it off forever.

CHAPTER 7

Why People Are Fat

If you want to get rich, write a book on how to lose weight. Americans are obsessed with losing weight. Yet Americans are among the fattest people in the world. Statistics vary, but at the moment, according to the Centers for Disease Control and Prevention, over 35 percent of Americans are *obese,* and nearly 70 percent are overweight. Still, we're doing more to lose weight, than ever. There are more diet books available than ever before. More people are on diets than ever before. More people drink diet sodas, eat diet, prepackaged food, and take diet pills than ever before. More people exercise than ever before. But the fact is, with all of the effort we've put into losing weight, as a nation, we're still *fatter* than ever before. Why is this?

Although rates of obesity have risen in other countries, the United States has had the distinction of being the *fattest country in the entire world* until recently, in 2013, when Mexico surpassed us to claim that honor.

First, we'll focus on the fundamentals so you can understand *why* you're overweight and how you've been lied to.

The United States government, through various agencies, has had a standard party line on the obesity epidemic. As I mentioned earlier in the book, "experts" state things as *fact* when, in reality, their statements are opinions, not facts. What the federal agencies say concerning obesity has constantly changed over time. Years ago the standard party line was the four basic food groups: **meat, dairy, grains, plus fruits and vegetables**. No one really questioned where those four basic food groups came from. I remember a food group poster in school back in the sixties. When I looked at it closely, I noticed that on the bottom it said that it was sponsored by the American Dairy Association. No wonder dairy products had their own food group. Isn't it surprising that the dairy association, whose only objective is to increase the consumption of dairy products (and thus profits), would strategically put a poster in school designed to brainwash kids into believing that in order to be healthy they had to eat dairy products at every meal? It's *always* been "*all about the money*."

> ...we'll focus on the fundamentals so you can understand why you're overweight and how you've been lied to.

The party line for obesity has always been, "If you want to lose weight you must eat fewer calories and exercise more." However, there are "experts" who claim to have "scientific proof" that calories are not the issue at all; it's *fat* that you must consume less of to lose weight. Then there are still *other* experts who have just as much scientific evidence to prove that fat is not the issue after all; the real culprit is carbohydrates. And yet *another* group of experts claim that "food combining" is the secret to losing weight. Then there's a long line of still more experts, each holding a stack of research espousing their so-called "fact" about losing weight: the glycemic index, insulin secretion, hormonal imbalances, genetics... the list goes on and on.

As I said in the beginning of the book, no one really knows anything when it comes to medicine, health, disease, illness, sickness, or obesity. We all look at studies, general observations, personal experiences, other people's anecdotes, and we come up with conclusions that make the most sense to us. However, why one person is fat and another skinny, no one really knows. Everyone is just presenting a theory, including me. I'm going to present my theory as to why you're fat, and I'm going to explain a system that will allow you to lose weight easier than ever before and keep it off once and for all. I could, as everyone else does, present my information as the absolute gospel truth, and though I believe that it *is*, it would be arrogant to say so. As I've done before, I'll preface my theory by saying that "it is based on the information I have at the time. As more information becomes available my theory may be altered, or improved." With that said, let's look at something we all know is true.

Everyone reading this knows someone who does not exercise; who eats huge amounts of food, including the so-called fattening foods like pizza, pasta, ice cream, cookies, and cakes—you name it, they eat it. We all know someone like this who, nonetheless, is as skinny as a rail and never gains a pound.

When I was growing up my own brother could eat anything he wanted, in any amount, at any time of the day, and he **Never Gained Any Weight.** If I'd eaten the same amount and did exactly the same things he did in terms of exercise, I would have blown up to 300 pounds.

Some people's bodies seem genetically designed to be thin, while other's bodies seem genetically destined to be fat. At least that's how it appears. However, I was looking through history books about Nazi concentration camps in World War II and noticed that the people behind the barbed wire were *all* skinny. There were no fat people there. I wondered if some of those people were genetically predisposed to be thin and others predisposed to be fat. I wondered if those who made it out of the concentration camps and went back to their normal routines, remained thin and other people, because of their genetic predisposition, got fatter. The point is it doesn't make a difference what your genetic predisposition is; if you're not eating any food for a long period of time, you're going to get skinny. But that doesn't answer the question about why a person in America is more likely to be fat than a person in another country.

Based on personal experience, thousands of scientific papers, and interviews with thousands of people in nearly every state in over a fifteen-year period, I've come up with some interesting conclusions about why people, Americans in particular, are fat.

1. **Most fat people have a low metabolism.**
    This means that you can eat some food and even if you eat a small amount your body won't burn it off very quickly. Instead, it turns into fat. If you had a high metabolism you could eat large amounts of food and it wouldn't turn to fat in your body. So, the number one reason a person is fat is because of a low metabolism.

    Why is this so specific to America, (and Mexico, apparently) as opposed to other countries? I will explain. But first, what exactly is metabolism? In simple terms, there are certain organs and glands in the body that regulate how your body burns food for fuel and how it converts food into fat. These include the thyroid, pancreas, liver, stomach, small and large intestines, and colon. When you have a slow metabolism, there's a good chance that some of these organs and glands are not working at optimal levels. Always remember, if you find a problem where the body is not operating as it is supposed to, you have to ask the question, "What caused that not to operate properly?" You must always look for the cause first.

There are many causes for low metabolism, including yo-yo dieting. If you've repeatedly lost and gained weight I can tell you that your metabolism is all screwed up.

So, let's look at each one of these reasons, and find out what caused the malfunction.

o **Most Fat People Have an Under-active Thyroid.**
   If you have an under-active thyroid (called a hypoactive thyroid), your body's ability to convert food to energy is slow, and the likelihood that the food you eat will turn into fat is greater than usual. What is the number one cause of a hypoactive thyroid? There's no consensus. But it appears that one contributing factor is the fluoride in the water that you drink. Fluoride is not added to drinking water in most other countries. This is *one* of the reasons Americans have such a high propensity for an under-active thyroid, a low metabolism, and being overweight. Bear in mind it's just *one* contributing factor. There's no one thing that causes obesity; it's a number of things

o **Most Fat People Have a Pancreas that Does Not Work Properly.**
   The pancreas secretes insulin. Fat people appear to have a pancreas that secretes insulin at a faster rate than thin people. A fat person's pancreas also secretes more insulin than that of a thin person. What causes the pancreas to secrete more insulin at a faster rate? The answer: No one really knows. But based on the information we have, it appears to be caused by some of the chemical additives contained in the food served in America. Many of these food additives are not put in food in other countries. It also appears that the large amounts of refined sugar cause this pancreatic problem as well. America's food has more

processed sugar and high fructose corn syrup than food in other countries.

o **Most Fat People Have a Clogged and Sluggish Liver.** The liver is a detoxifying organ. When it's clogged, your metabolism slows down. What causes the liver to clog up? The number one reason your liver is not operating properly is the nonprescription and prescription drugs you've taken throughout your life. Most notably, if you take cholesterol reducing drugs, your liver is definitely clogged. Chlorine and fluoride in the water is another cause of a clogged liver. Chemical additives in processed food, fast food and animal fats clog the liver. Refined sugar, high fructose corn syrup and white flour clog the liver. Artificial sweeteners, monosodium glutamate, and preservatives clog the liver. The bottom line is the pharmaceutical companies clog your liver and the publicly traded food industry clogs your liver.

o **Most Fat People Have A Sluggish Digestive System** Overweight people seem to have a problem producing digestive enzymes. If you're not producing enough digestive enzymes your food doesn't get converted into energy and there's a higher chance it will be stored as fat. What's the reason for not producing enough digestive enzymes? It appears to be the chemical additives that are in the American food supply. The small and large intestines of overweight people are generally not as healthy as those of thin people. What is the cause of this? Candida yeast overgrowth. Why would someone have a yeast overgrowth? Antibiotics. Antibiotics kill all of the friendly bacteria in the intestines, which allow Candida (the unfriendly bacteria) to proliferate in the digestive system. This slows digestion and elimination.

So, if we were to ask *what is the number one reason for a slow metabolism*, the answer would be: "What you put in your body." The poisons you put in your body affect your metabolism. These toxins include: nonprescription and prescription drugs, chemical pesticides used in the process of growing food, artificial food additives, and the chemicals added to our water, primarily chlorine and fluoride.

There's another reason your metabolism is low. It has to do with exercise. The more muscle you have, the higher your metabolism. Americans, by and large, tend not to have a lot of muscle in their bodies. This means that calories aren't burned as effectively as they could be. The second most important issue in relation to exercise is sitting too much and walking too little. The human body is designed to walk. A study of thin Europeans, Africans, Chinese, and South Americans showed that the common denominator amongst the lean subjects in the study was the amount of walking they did daily. People who walk a lot every day tend to be thin. People who walk less than a tenth of a mile per day tend to be overweight.

2. **The majority of people who are overweight eat when they're not hungry.**
   This is caused by two factors: (a) emotional eating, or (b) physiological food cravings. Emotional eating is triggered by stress or stressful situations. Physiological food cravings are generally caused by the toxins you put in your body, or Candida yeast overgrowth.

3. **Most fat people have a large appetite.**
   If you're overweight you probably find yourself hungry a lot of the time. The hunger is generally caused by the body's inability to assimilate nutrients due to lack of digestive enzymes and Candida yeast overgrowth. Another reason you're hungry is that certain food additives increase hunger.

4. **Most fat people have hormonal imbalances.**

   If you're overweight, statistics show there's a high likelihood that your body is secreting too much of certain hormones and not enough of others. This imbalance is generally caused by excess toxins in the body and by a sedentary lifestyle.

5. **Most fat people eat larger portions than thin people.**

   This is caused by a combination of things: larger appetite, inability to assimilate nutrients, physiological cravings, stress, emotional issues, and the increase in the size of portions packaged and sold by the food industry. In Europe, for example, candy bars and snack food come in packages that are smaller than American-sized portions. Restaurants in Europe serve portions 30 to 40 percent smaller than their American counterparts.

6. **Fat people consume more "diet food."**

   Here is a major mind blower. Most diet food actually makes you fatter. Diet products, i.e. those labeled: "diet," "low-fat," "sugar-free," "low-calorie," "light," "low-carb," "lean," etc., are filled with either artificial sweeteners, high levels of sugar (added to low-fat foods), or chemical additives that make you fatter, not thinner. This is the dirty little secret the food industry does not want you to know. These additives can increase your appetite and make you physically addicted to the food, causing you to gain weight.

7. **Most fat people's bodies are highly toxic.**

   Toxins lodge primarily in the colon and fat cells throughout the body. When the body is high in toxins it retains water and increases its fat stores in an effort to dilute the poisons.

8. **Most fat people eat before they go to bed.**

   When you sleep, your metabolism slows considerably. When you eat late at night, food doesn't get a chance to burn off and it converts to fat easier.

9. **Most fat people are affected by the growth hormone put in meat and dairy products.**

   Our meat and dairy supply is loaded with growth hormones. These hormones are given to the animals to speed their growth in order to increase production and profits. When you consume nonorganic meat and dairy you're also consuming growth hormones. This contributes to obesity, and it's also one of the reasons children today are maturing earlier and earlier.

10. **Most fat people see themselves as fat.**

    Remember Earl Nightingale's discovery, "The Strangest Secret"? After years of research he discovered that *people become what they think about.* Fat people constantly think about their weight, thus creating the undesired result.

The dirty little secret the food industry doesn't want you to know.

Here I am blowing the whistle on what I believe to be one of the greatest, most devious lies in American history. The food industry consists of publicly traded corporations. These companies have one objective: To increase profits. The only way a food company can increase profits is to produce their products at the lowest possible cost and sell them at the highest possible price, and sell as much of them as they can.

The people running the food companies, the officers and directors, do not care about the health and wellbeing of the American public. They care only about the profits. You may have a hard time understanding or believing just how greedy these people can be. Did you know that there are a number of billionaires in prisons around the world? Why? Because the more money they make, the more money they need to make. For many of these people it becomes an addiction. Some of the officers and directors of food companies are so consumed with making more money they'll do anything, and knowingly hurt anybody, including you, just to make more money. It's sad, but true.

When the executives of food companies think only about how to increase profits, and they need to come up with ways to make their product (food) cheaper, those ways include genetic engineering the food and spraying chemical poisons on it, so that the crops won't be damaged by disease or bugs. The soil is loaded with chemicals to make the plants grow faster, the animals are pumped full of growth hormone to make them grow faster. These companies will do anything to get their products produced less expensively. They also want to sell these products at the highest possible price, and they want to sell massive amounts of them. So here's what happens. In making their products faster and cheaper, they become highly toxic. If you've ever been in a mass production facility you would be appalled at how food is "made."

These food companies must also be sure that you continue to buy and eat more food. They have laboratories where thousands of chemical additives are researched and tested. These laboratories are in secret locations with tighter security than the CIA headquarters. The objective is to make the food physically addictive, to make it increase your appetite, and to make it cause you to gain weight. Two common additives that appear to do this include the artificial sweetener aspartame and the sweetener high fructose corn syrup. Like the tobacco industry, the executives of the food industry vehemently deny these allegations. Remember, the tobacco industry denied knowingly making cigarettes physically addictive.

The fact is the American food supply will make you fat no matter what you do. This is why when thin people from other countries come to America, they seem to gain weight even though it appears that they're not eating any differently than they had previously.

When first lady Michelle Obama began encouraging people to exercise more and eat healthier food, some politicians actually railed against this. Some even suggested that Obama was endangering people and blaming an increase in pedestrian deaths on her campaign to get people to walk more. How likely do you think it is that some of those same politicians had financial ties to the food industry? The food industry is so profit driven it does not want people to eat less and get fit! The food industry wants you fat and eating more and more food every year.

This is the reason diet products in the form of pills, powders, food bars, and prepackaged diet foods will never work. The good news is that knowing the truth allows you to take simple steps to lose weight faster and easier than ever before. This knowledge also allows you to eat the foods you enjoy, never deprive yourself, and stay thin for life.

CHAPTER 8

How to Lose Weight Effortlessly and Keep It Off

I struggled with my weight for much of my life. I was a fat kid. I tried every diet, every weight loss pill, and I even hired a personal trainer, exercising as much as five hours a day. Whatever I lost, I put right back on. While I was losing weight I was hungry, tired, and grumpy. I never understood what the problem was, until I went overseas and found the answer. While living abroad I ate everything I wanted, and yet I began to lose weight without even trying. This led me to the discovery of the reasons why Americans are so overweight, and it showed me an easy, workable solution.

Though this isn't a explicitly a weight loss book (for more weight loss suggestions, listen to my book on CD, *Weight Loss Secrets "They" Don't Want You to Know About* which you can find at www. NaturalCuresBook.com if you don't already have it), I *am* going to give you a list of simple steps that will help you lose weight and keep it off once and for all. Many readers have implemented the recommendations that follow with great success. You may have heard some of their stories in my infomercial. I can assure you that following these steps will turn your body into a fat-burning furnace and bring your weight to its ideal place. These steps have tremendous health benefits as well.

1. **Drink a glass of water immediately upon arising.**
   This starts the body's metabolism and cleansing. Ideally, the water should be distilled, no tap water, and it should be room temperature or slightly warm, not cold. For an added boost, squeeze some lemon into the water. Warm water aids digestion. And the lemon stimulates the liver and aids in detoxification. And for even *more* of a boost, add a dash of cayenne pepper. The hot pepper detoxifies, boosts blood flow, and helps with weight loss.

2. **Drink eight glasses of distilled water each day.**
   People think drinking water will make them bloated. The exact opposite is true. If you're overweight you need to flush the toxins from your fat cells. Water, and lots of it, is absolutely needed to lose weight.

3. **Eat a big breakfast.**
   Many overweight people eat a small breakfast, or none at all, and then eat large amounts later in the day. This is not a good approach for weight loss or weight maintenance. You'll lose more weight if you make breakfast a large meal and dinner a lighter meal. Your breakfast should consist of as much as you want of the following items (everything should be organic): apples, pears, berries, kiwis, pineapples, grapefruit, plums, peaches, prunes, figs, raw butter (raw means not pasteurized or homogenized), raw milk, plain yogurt (this means no sugar or added fruit), wild smoked salmon, beef in any form as long as it's organic, chicken in any form as long as it's organic, lamb in any form as long as it's organic, tuna, sardines, eggs, tomatoes, peppers, salsa,

celery, carrots, any green leafy vegetables, potatoes (preferably sweet potatoes) in limited amounts, coffee in limited amounts made with pure water (not tap water) with raw milk or cream and raw honey (in small amounts) or stevia as a sweetener, and organic tea (no pesticides). Notice what is *not* on this list? Anything made with flour or wheat. Bagels, toast, donuts, etc. Limit refined carbohydrates.

4. **Eat organic grapefruit all day.**
   Remember the grapefruit diet? Well, it turns out that there actually *is* an enzyme in grapefruit that burns fat. Eating grapefruits all day, as many and as often as you desire, will speed the fat burning process.

5. **Eat organic apples all day.**
   The old saying is true: An apple a day keeps the doctor away. Apples are loaded with fiber and nutrients; they normalize the blood sugar and decrease appetite. You should eat at least one organic apple every day.

6. **Eat a huge salad at lunch and dinner.**
   Use a few cups of fresh organic leafy greens as the base of your meal. Leafy greens include romaine, spinach, kale, arugula, Swiss chard, and others. Iceberg lettuce does not count. If you do make it your base, you can add other organic vegetables and some lean protein and even a grain, like brown rice or quinoa. For dressing, use olive oil and lemon and lime, or organic vinegar. If you really want to speed the weight loss process, use organic apple cider vinegar. Add some organic Himalayan pink sea salt, fresh ground pepper, or some garlic for taste. Do not use processed salad dressings from the supermarket. They will contain chemicals and often sugar or high fructose corn syrup as well. If you *don't* make salad the meal, at least eat a huge salad *along with* your meal. I don't care if your lunch is a cheeseburger

and french fries (as long as it's organic), eat a huge salad first and you'll be amazed by how you lose weight.

7. **Eat only organic meat, poultry, and fish.**

   One of the reasons you are overweight is because of the growth hormones put in meat and poultry. If you want to lose weight, eat as much meat and poultry as you like as long as it is organic, grass fed, ideally kosher, and most importantly, has not been given growth hormones. The fish you eat should not be farm raised.

8. **Eat hot peppers.**

   Anything spicy or hot will increase your metabolism and make you burn fat quicker. Imagine for breakfast having some scrambled eggs, some lamb chops, and some chopped peppers. Smother the eggs with some organic hot salsa and you will simply lose weight faster.

9. **Use organic apple cider vinegar.**

   Take a couple of teaspoons of organic apple cider vinegar in a cup of distilled water before meals and you'll be amazed at how your clothes will become bigger in no time. This vinegar suppresses the appetite and also lowers blood sugar levels. It promotes the secretion of hydrochloric acid in the stomach, which promotes good digestion and better assimilation of nutrients. I don't recommend daily use because the acid can be harmful to tooth enamel and high levels can lead to reduced bone density. But using it a couple of times a week is beneficial and will aid weight loss without harmful effects.

10. **Consume organic extra virgin coconut oil.**

    Specifically, replace the cooking oil you've been using with coconut oil. (Olive oil is fine, but stop using soybean oil, corn oil, lard or processed butter.) Coconut oil erroneously got a bad reputation years ago when it was believed that because it's a saturated fat, it clogged the arteries. It's not true. Coconut oil has no cholesterol and it does not affect the body in the same way that saturated animal fat does. The other great thing about coconut oil is that it gives the metabolism a boost, so it aids in weight loss. Don't go crazy with it, because it's still high in calories. But if you use coconut oil in place of other oil, it will help you lose weight. It tastes good enough that you can also use it in place of butter on vegetables, or baked potatoes.

11. **Consume probiotics.**

Probiotic foods are fermented foods. Rich in enzymes, they help the body's digestive system by breaking down sugars. They also help us absorb more nutrients from our food. They promote good bacteria in the intestines and minimize bad bacteria (like Candida). They assist with weight loss by destroying bile salts in the intestines, which reduce the absorption of fat calories. Some probiotic foods you should add to your diet are: plain organic yogurt, kimchi, miso, sauerkraut, pickles and tempeh.

12. **Do not eat after six p.m.**

This takes some getting used to, so do the best you can. If you follow it, you'll be amazed at how much easier it is to lose weight when you stop eating at this hour. I know it's not easy, but the good news is you can eat *well* during the day, and if you stop eating by 6:00 p.m., you'll still lose weight.

13. **Limit dairy products.**

If you are going to consume milk, cheese, butter, or any dairy products, eat only organic ones that have not been pasteurized or homogenized. The dairy products should be labeled "organic and raw." It may be hard to find raw dairy products in some parts of the country. The next best option is organic, not homogenized, but that has been pasteurized. Your last option is organic that has been both pasteurized and homogenized. Ideally, if you want to lose weight, reduce dairy regardless of what you're getting. Avoid milk, cream, cheese and ice cream. Plain yogurt (preferably Greek) is good and does aid weight loss, because the live cultures assist the digestive system. Definitely do not consume any dairy products that are not organic because they will have growth hormones in them which will slow your weight loss.

14. **No white sugar, white flour, or white rice.**
    White sugar is addictive and makes you fat. Use unprocessed sweeteners in small amounts, preferably raw, organic honey, organic coconut sugar, or stevia extract. White flour, as I've mentioned previously, when mixed with water, makes paste. It does the same thing in your body. Eating white flour clogs up your digestive system and slows your metabolism, which keeps you from losing weight. Use organic whole grain flours that have not been processed or stripped of the fiber, or even better, eat whole grains in place of flour-based products. Oatmeal, quinoa and brown rice are good choices. Avoid white rice. White rice is stripped of its fiber and it spikes blood sugar levels, which leads to inflammation.

15. **No wheat.**
    The wheat produced in this country is genetically modified to the point wherein it isn't the same grain it was originally. This "Frankenwheat" is addictive and it irritates the digestive system. This is not exclusive to people who are gluten sensitive. No one should eat wheat. Removing wheat from you diet is one of the best things you can do to lose weight. This means eliminating most bread. This means eliminating pasta. I know that's hard, and will take some getting used to, but replace it with other grains like oatmeal, brown rice and quinoa and you will get used to it.

16. **No diet sodas or diet food.**

    Diet sodas actually make you fat. They're loaded with chemicals that reek havoc on your metabolism. I did an experiment with people who drank diet soft drinks on a regular basis. For two weeks they replaced their diet soda with regular soda. Amazingly, though they were ingesting more calories from the sugar-sweetened soda, no one gained any weight. Even more shocking was that 80 percent of the people actually lost weight. This is *not* an invitation to go drink a bunch of regular soda—I don't advocate that (all sodas are bad for you), but I want you to see how you're being duped as a consumer. Diet sodas are promoted so heavily, because they're cheaper to make than regular sodas, and because the product is so physically addictive it's been called the "new crack." There is simply no benefit to drinking diet soda. It's the same scam with diet *foods*. Don't eat them. They're not healthy and they're full of chemicals that will actually make it more difficult for you to lose weight. Eat real, wholesome food.

17. **No aspartame or ANY artificial sweeteners.**

    Aspartame, which goes by the name NutraSweet®, will make you fat. All other artificial sweeteners, including saccharin, Splenda®, or anything else, should be avoided. These are toxins. I encourage you to *release* toxins, not store them up in your body. Aspartame triggers food cravings (for sugar and carbohydrates), which obviously works *against* weight loss efforts. And it's addictive. If you use it, you'll tend to use it a lot. Don't even start. Stevia is okay, depending on the brand. Don't buy the kind sold in major grocery stores masquerading as stevia. Truvia is *not* stevia, despite the claims. Look at the ingredients. If it lists a lot of chemicals, avoid it. There are good brands of liquid stevia available online containing just stevia extract, vegetable glycerin, and a small amount of alcohol.

18. **No monosodium glutamate.**

Monosodium glutamate (MSG) is an excitotoxin, which means it over stimulates the cells until it kills them. It makes you fat; it can cause all kinds of medical problems (including fibromyalgia), and it can affect your mood making you depressed. It can also be physically addictive. Unfortunately, the food industry has lobbied Congress to pass laws allowing monosodium glutamate to be added to food while not being listed on the label. There are dozens of words such as spices, natural flavoring, hydrolyzed vegetable protein, etc., that are in fact MSG in disguise. This is why I recommend buying organic, where everything in the ingredient list is something you recognize and can pronounce. Also, MSG is in virtually all fast food, including things you would never imagine, like pizza. This is why people in other countries seem to be able to eat all kinds of food without gaining weight. It's not just the food, but the ingredients used in American food processing that keeps us fat.

19. **No high fructose corn syrup.**

This sweetener, like many of the items on this list, makes you fat and it's physically addictive. I know a woman who lost 15 pounds by doing nothing other than removing high fructose corn syrup from her diet. This corn-derived poison has been linked to obesity, hypertension, and diabetes among other problems. Never ever consume it. In fact, just stop buying *any* processed foods, because it is in nearly all of them. Read the labels on the food you buy. You'll be shocked by how ubiquitous high fructose corn syrup is. But once you realize this, and you see how it's added to so many products, you'll be empowered to make better choices and cook your own food.

20. **No fast food or chain restaurants.**

Any chain or franchise restaurant that sells fast food produces it in such a way that it will make you fat. You can actually eat French fries and cheeseburgers and lose weight, provided that the ingredients you use are organic. It's virtually impossible to eat food in a chain or franchise restaurant where the food has *not* been processed to last for years, which means it is full of preservatives. In addition to that there are chemicals added to make the food taste great, get you physically addicted to it, increase your appetite and make you fatter. Remember, these are businesses whose main objective is to make a profit. If the food tastes amazing, gets you physically addicted, increases your appetite, and makes you fat, the restaurant is guaranteed success. They're like drug dealers getting their customers hooked and continually coming back for more. This is the sad truth of what's happening in our food industry today.

21. **Take digestive enzymes.**

There's an excellent chance your body is not producing enough digestive enzymes if you're gaining weight, feeling bloated, and have gas, indigestion, and/or constipation. Go to your health food store and inquire, or do an online search. Try a few kinds to see which one works best for you.

22. **Get fifteen colonics in thirty days.**

This process will clean your colon, making it easier for your body to assimilate nutrients. This reduces hunger, it reduces cravings, and increases metabolism. Colonics also allow your body to digest food faster so that it will not turn to fat.

23. **Do a colon cleanse.**

If you do the fifteen colonics, you won't need a colon cleanse, but if you *don't* do the colonics, you should do one. If you're significantly overweight, your digestive system is more than likely sluggish. You should be moving your bowels *at least* once daily, preferably more. Cleansing the colon will help with weight loss, dramatically increase your metabolism, and benefit your body by eliminating toxins. There are many colon-cleansing programs available. Inquire at your local health food store for recommendations, or research them online.

24. **Do a Candida cleanse.**

If you're overweight, you most certainly have a Candida yeast overgrowth, probably throughout your entire body. Losing weight will be difficult and slow and keeping it off nearly impossible as long as this condition persists. If you wipe out the excess Candida, losing weight will be much easier and keeping it off will be easier, too. There is plenty of information about Candida cleanses online.

25. **Do a liver cleanse.**

If you are overweight your liver is most definitely clogged and needs attention. The liver is one of our most important detox organs. Cleansing the liver will assist it in detoxifying the body's waste, which in turn will help the digestive system process food more efficiently so that you can lose weight more easily. There are many liver cleanses on the market. Research them and see what works best for you. In the meantime, you can help begin the liver cleansing process by eating lots of fresh leafy greens, omitting sugar and food high in animal fats, and drinking distilled water with lemon or with lemon and cayenne pepper first thing every morning.

26. **Fast**

This is intimidating to most people, and it can be difficult, but the benefits are so fantastic I urge you to do it. It will change your body and your life. A twenty-one day organic juice fast will completely detoxify your body, flush out your fat cells, and reset your body's weight set point. It will also leave you thinner, revitalized and feeling like a new (improved) person. Ideally, you should have a juicer and juice the organic fruits and vegetables yourself, emphasizing leafy greens as the base for most of your juices. Organic juice fasting lets the digestive system heal itself by cleansing it and giving it a rest. The first few days are challenging, but it becomes easier and you will soon feel energized. Not only will you shed weight, but some people experience increased wellbeing, more clarity in their thoughts, and an improvement in emotional health. One caveat: a fast that's longer than a few days should be done under the supervision of a professional healthcare provider.

27. **Use infrared saunas.**

Infrared saunas increase metabolism, dramatically reduce toxins, speed weight loss, and burn fat. Ideally they're used on a daily basis, but I realize this is impractical for most people. Do the best you can. Spas and gyms are slowly catching on about the benefits of infrared saunas over traditional saunas, so they're getting easier to find in most big cities.

28. **Add muscle.**

Muscle burns fat. When you add muscle through exercise you're increasing your body's metabolism. Weight training is probably the method you're most familiar with. It's not the method I prefer, but it's better than not adding muscle. The reason it's not my preference is because I believe that it builds muscle in a way that blocks energy rather than allowing it to flow through your body. Blocked energy is not ideal. In my opinion, the best way to add muscle without blocking energy is to do exercises that add muscle, while also stretching the body and keeping it limber. Consider yoga, Pilates, ballet, swimming, or martial arts.

29. **Walk for at least one hour, nonstop, per day.**

The body is designed to walk. Research shows that slow, rhythmic movement exercise, like walking, resets the body's weight set point and creates a leaner physique. A one-hour walk every day will change your body dramatically in as little as one month.

30. **Rebound.**

Using a rebounder, or mini-trampoline, stimulates and strengthens every cell in the body simultaneously. Gently jumping up and down on a rebounder for just ten minutes a day stimulates the lymphatic system and increases your metabolism. It is very effective for weight loss and enhances overall health.

31. **Practice deep breathing.**

Oxygen breaks down and burns fat. Most people do not breathe deeply enough to stimulate their metabolism and fat burning capabilities. Fat is made up of oxygen, hydrogen and carbon. When the oxygen we breathe reaches fat molecules it breaks them down into carbon dioxide and water. The blood then picks up the carbon dioxide and returns it to the lungs and we exhale it. So the more oxygen you use, the more fat you'll burn. Breathe deeply, using your diaphragm. While breathing *alone* won't transform your body (sorry, you still have to exercise!), deep breathing will help tremendously. Try doing it when you wake up, before you go to bed and even occasionally while you're working or waiting in line somewhere. Take in a deep breath, hold it a moment and exhale slowly, then repeat. Do this at least five times and build up to ten times or more. Consider deep breathing while you do your daily activities; it will increase the benefits.

32. **Wear magnetic finger rings.**

Special magnetic rings worn on the little finger of each hand while you sleep can have amazing results. Magnetic rings help speed the metabolism. They also assist with fluid retention.

33. **Cheat once in a while.**

You want ice cream, cookies, cakes, chocolate, French fries, pizza, potato chips? Don't completely deprive yourself. It's better to eat a little something without guilt than not eat it and feel bad about it. Not eating food and being stressed about it can make you fat, because after a while, you'll rebel and binge to the point where your eating will be out of control. Allow yourself a little bit of whatever it is you're craving. If you follow my recommendations, the boost you'll get from how wonderful your weight loss looks will help you change your eating habits. When you start omitting processed foods, you'll stop craving them, because the chemicals that keep you addicted will be out of your system. Ideally, if you *are* going to cheat and want cookies, cakes, ice cream, potato chips, etc., don't buy these products from the supermarket. Go to a health food store and buy the natural or organic counterpart. The advantage is that if you choose wisely, you can enjoy these treats without all of the processing and chemicals that make and keep you fat.

34. **Reduce or eliminate the "uncontrollable" urge to eat when you're not hungry.**

If you're an emotional eater and have uncontrollable urges and compulsions to eat when you're not hungry you may benefit from hypnosis. Look for a licensed hypnotherapist. You may also benefit from a process called "tapping." Look into the Emotional Freedom Technique (EFT) or Thought Field Therapy (TRT). Both employ tapping and can be used to eliminate compulsions. I recommend the book *Tapping The Healer Within: How to Instantly Conquer Fears, Anxieties, and Emotional Distress* by Roger Callahan.

It's amazing that little things can make a difference. When looking at this list, a good way to attack it is to pick one thing on the list and do that for a few days. Then, look for another thing on the list and while still doing the first thing, add the second. Do that until you feel comfortable adding something else. These techniques absolutely work and they will not only help you lose weight, but they'll benefit your health overall.

And if you desire the ever-elusive toned tummy, try these approaches for a flatter stomach.

First, get enough rest. Studies show that people who sleep just six hours a night are 23% more likely to be obese than those who sleep seven to eight hours a night. "People with a lack of sleep suffer a condition known as leptin resistance," says Stephen Eddey, principal of Health Schools Australia. "Leptin is a hormone that is released from our fat cells and which suppresses appetite. If you're not getting enough sleep, your leptin fails to work properly and therefore your appetite increases."

Dehydration is possibly another reason why a flat belly can be elusive. That's because your body requires sufficient amounts of water to stay healthy. Without it, among other things, your stomach will tend to be bloated.

Plus, drinking enough water can help reduce food cravings. For example, a craving for carbohydrates and sugar can be a sign of dehydration. Since carbohydrates raise blood sugar levels which in turn increase blood flow to the brain, not having enough water in your body can create cravings.

CHAPTER 9

How to Read Food Labels

Hopefully by now you're convinced that there most definitely *are* toxic chemicals in the majority of the food you purchase in major supermarkets, or eat in most fast food restaurants. Our food supply is different than it was seventy-five, fifty, or even as recently as twenty-five years ago. Many of you eat the same brands and products today that you ate twenty or thirty years ago, without realizing that the product is no longer the same; it's been modified. Today that same product could contain a hundred times the number of chemical toxins that it contained twenty-five or fifty years ago. In an effort to produce food more cheaply, make it last longer, make you physically addicted to it, increase your appetite, and make you fat, food manufacturers process and load their products with chemicals that add toxins and destroy the living enzymes. This wipes out much of the food's nutritional value.

The bottom line is that today it's nearly impossible to go to a supermarket or fast food restaurant and buy anything to eat or drink that's *not* full of chemicals, reduced in nutritional value, or energetically altered. Ideally, you would never eat in fast food restaurants, and never buy anything mass-produced by large food manufacturers. You'd buy *only* organic fruits, vegetables, nuts, seeds, grains, meats, eggs, and dairy products and make everything in your house from scratch. But, realistically, most of us can't do that, at least not all of the time. So is it a lost cause, or is there something you can do to eat food that has fewer toxins, more nutrition, and that hasn't been energetically altered? The answer is yes. It may not be perfect, but it'll be infinitely better than what you're doing now.

> Our food supply is different than it was seventy-five, fifty, or even as recently as twenty-five years ago.

When you go food shopping, **avoid major supermarkets**. When you shop for food, consider, instead, going to a farmer's market. Buy organic fruits, vegetables, nuts, grains, herbs and spices from small independent growers whom you can meet and talk with, so you can feel confident that what you're buying is actually good for you. In some areas there are "food co-ops" wherein members organize and make the decisions about what food is sold and where it comes from. I recommend these, because they're generally run by people with a sincere interest in bringing good quality food to their communities. If you live in a house with a yard, consider planting fruit trees, or a vegetable garden. Even if you live in an apartment, you can grow some vegetables (like tomatoes, mushrooms, carrots and radishes) in pots indoors, or on a terrace, or rooftop.

The most convenient way to shop for high quality food is go to a whole food or natural health food store where they sell organic products. When you go to these stores, you have a better chance of finding things that aren't loaded with toxins, or energetically altered, the way the products in regular supermarkets are. Keep in mind, though, that not everything they sell in these natural or whole food stores is good for you. Remember, it's always all about the money. In some cases, these stores are also publicly traded companies that have to make a profit, so you have to read the labels. The key to reading labels is not to read the front of the package. This is where the company does its advertising, and where the marketing department has spent millions of dollars researching what will make you think it is healthy so you'll buy it. Take the box, package or jar, (no cans—avoid canned food, because can linings have the toxin Bisphenol A in them) and look for the *ingredients list*. I'm going to give you the most important words you should look for and avoid. When you see these, do not buy that product. Just say *no*, and put it back.

1. **Anything You Can't Pronounce**

   If you can't pronounce the word, it's a chemical. They can call it anything they want. They can say that it comes from a plant, or that it's all natural. But it's not true. Keep in mind food manufacturers lobby Congress to get legislation passed that allows these food manufactures to call chemicals "all natural ingredients." Bottom line: if you can't pronounce it, don't buy it.

2. **Monosodium Glutamate**

   Never buy anything with monosodium glutamate (MSG) in it. MSG is an excitotoxin, which means it damages nerve cells. It's dangerous; it makes you fat, increases your appetite, and causes all types of physical and medical problems.

3. **Sugar**

   The sugar used in processed food is refined, which means they've taken natural sugarcane and turned it into a drug. It's added to food for its sweetness, but also for its chemically addictive qualities. It is also laced with the chemicals used in growing sugarcane. Avoid it entirely.

4. **High Fructose Corn Syrup**

This corn derived, toxic sweetener is highly addictive, and makes you fat. It can lead to plaque buildup and narrowing of the arteries. It also contributes to fat deposits in your liver.

5. **Aspartame**

This sweetener is an excitotoxin, which, like MSG, can damage nerve cells. It makes you fat, it makes you hungry, it makes you depressed, and it leads to all types of medical conditions including PMS, chronic fatigue syndrome, fibromyalgia, and migraines.

6. **Dextrose**

This is a chemically made sweetener. It's a simple carbohydrate, a source of "empty calories" and consuming it can lead to weight gain.

7. **Sucralose-Splenda®**

This chemical sweetener is poisonous and makes you fat. It was produced so that the food industry could capitalize on the low-carbohydrate craze. Now, products can have "no- carbohydrates" or "low-carbohydrates" and still taste sweet. The problem is that it's artificial, and these man-made sweeteners do in fact increase your appetite, make you depressed, cause all types of symptoms (including migraine headaches, PMS, depression, fibromyalgia, and allergies), and most importantly, make you fat.

8. **Artificial Color**

Stay away from food dyes. They're chemical poisons. Many of the food dyes in American products are acknowledged to be toxic and banned elsewhere in the world. Some of the dyes can cause a list of health problems including tumors, chromosomal damage, hyperactivity, insomnia, aggression and violent behavior, eczema, hives, asthma and others. Anything that has food dye in it is processed, so avoid it.

9. **Natural and Artificial Flavors**

If it says "natural" or "artificial flavors" on the label, know that this is where lobbyists have done a magnificent job of allowing the food industry to deceive the public. "Natural flavor" is not natural at all and is no better, nor much different from "artificial flavor." Much of the food in today's high-tech processing is so altered that it loses most of its flavor. Consequently, food manufacturers must add chemicals (natural and/or artificial flavors) to make the food taste like it's supposed to. If you were to ask the food companies to individually list the ingredients in "natural" and/or "artificial" flavors, they would refuse. My insiders tell me that if they did reveal that list, the ingredients for both natural and artificial flavors would contain hundreds of chemicals. While a single chemical may not have major immediate negative effects, when you combine two, three, or four of these chemicals, just like in chemistry class, new chemicals are formed. What these new chemicals do is dangerous for the body. Avoid anything with natural and/or artificial flavors on the label.

10. **Spices**

Be wary when a label says "spices" without specifying what those spices are. More than likely they are *not* merely spices, they also contain chemicals. *Real* spices are great, but if the spices in the product were in fact *real*, they would be able to name them. "Spices" fall under a category similar to natural flavors.

11. **Hydrogenated Oil or Partially Hydrogenated Oil**

If it's hydrogenated or partially hydrogenated, don't buy it. It's a trans fat. Trans fats cause heart disease, make you fat, and can lead to a whole host of other medical conditions.

12. **Palm Oil**

A deadly oil that's cheap to manufacture, and causes all types of physical problems. In its oxidized state, which is how it would appear in most foods, palm oil can threaten physiological and biochemical functions of the body. The dangers include toxicity to the heart, kidney, liver and lungs.

13. **Enriched Bleached Wheat Flour and Enriched Bleached White Flour**

Wheat production and processing in this country has unfortunately ruined it to the point wherein I don't recommend that you eat *any* product made from wheat or wheat flour. No bread, pasta, bagels, muffins, biscuits or cereals—*nothing* made of wheat will do your body any good. I know this is difficult to hear, but it's true. Sadly, wheat is now a toxin. Today's wheat is simply not the same product it was years ago. It was changed in order to make it stronger, and to make it grow better and faster. Wheat now contains sodium azide, which is a known toxin. It also contains new proteins that aren't found in the original version of wheat. Our bodies don't have the enzymes to break down these proteins and so they are impossible to digest. You've probably heard a lot about *gluten intolerance* over the past few years. Gluten is a protein composite that many people can't digest, hence the proliferation of "gluten free" products. But what you may not know is that *no one can properly digest gluten*. Though you may not experience the symptoms of the gluten intolerant, virtually all of us experience systemic inflammation from eating wheat. On top of that, wheat products contain a morphine-like compound that makes them highly addictive.

14. **Soy Protein Isolate**

This is a common toxic ingredient in protein shakes and protein bars. Stay away from it. You will never see organic soy protein isolate. The reason is that hexane, which is a petroleum solvent similar to gasoline, is often used to process soy protein isolate. The residues of chemicals like hexane remain in the food, but they're never listed on the label.

There you have the main things to stay away from. A good rule of thumb, however, is to read the labels. You may find things not included on this list that you should avoid. If the ingredients you see are not things that you could have in your own kitchen, or if the food is something you couldn't make yourself, stay away from it; it's dangerous.

Now I'd like to point out in greater detail just how different the food from a regular supermarket is compared to its equivalent purchased at a local health food store. Keep in mind that these products may seem nearly identical, but the differences are these: The food from the health food store will have fewer ingredients, the ingredients will be (mostly) organic, and there will be fewer chemicals in the food or no chemicals at all. The food hasn't been stripped of its nutritional value, and it hasn't been energetically destroyed.

> Keep in mind that most food producers want you to crave their food so you'll eat more of it.

The food from the health food store also tastes better because it's made with whole food ingredients. When you eat it you don't get constipation, bloating, or gas. Most people eat less because the nutrients are greater and more easily assimilated so you don't crave as much. Keep in mind that most food producers want you to crave their food so you'll eat more of it. That's how they increase their profits. Bottom line is the food from the health food store, generally, will have more nutrition, will have nothing energetically destroyed, will taste better, and have virtually no toxins in it. So let's go through a few products and note the differences on the labels.

A. Pancake Syrup

Health Food Store

Product name: Organic maple syrup

Ingredients: 100 percent raw, unprocessed, unfiltered maple syrup

Supermarket

Product name: Aunt Jemima Original Syrup

Ingredients: Corn syrup, high fructose corn syrup, water, cellulose gum, caramel color, salt, sodium benzoate, ascorbic acid, artificial flavors, natural flavors, sodium hexametaphosphate

B. Potato Chips

Health Food Store

Product name: Potato chips

Ingredients: Organic potatoes, organic sunflower oil, sea salt

Supermarket

Product name: Pringles Potato Chips

Ingredients: Dried potatoes, corn oil, cottonseed oil, sunflower oil, yellow corn meal, wheat starch, maltodextrin, salt, dextrose, whey, buttermilk, dried tomato, dried garlic, partially hydrogenated soybean oil, monosodium glutamate, corn syrup solids, dried onion, sodium casonate, multicacid, spices, annatto extract, modified corn starch, natural flavors, artificial flavors, disodium inosinate, disodium guanylate

C. Mayonnaise

Health Food Store

Product name: Organic mayonnaise

Ingredients: Expeller pressed soybean oil, organic whole eggs, water, organic egg yolks, organic honey, organic white vinegar, sea salt, organic dry mustard, organic lemon juice concentrate

Supermarket

Product name: Miracle Whip Mayonnaise

Ingredients: Water, soybean oil, vinegar, high fructose corn syrup, eggs, sugar, modified food starch, salt, mustard flower, artificial color, potassium sorbate, paprika, spices, natural flavors, dried garlic

D. Salad Dressing
Health Food Store
Product name: Salad dressing
Ingredients: Water, expeller pressed canola oil, balsamic vinegar, vine-ripened dried tomatoes, sea salt, garlic, oregano, basil, parsley, black pepper
Supermarket
Product name: Kraft Fat Free Salad Dressing
Ingredients: Water, tomato paste, high fructose corn syrup, vinegar, corn syrup, water, chopped pickles, modified food starch, salt, maltodextrin, soybean oil, egg yolks, xanthan gum, artificial color, mustard flower, potassium sorbate, calcium disodium, EDTA, phosphoric acid, dried onions, guar gum, spices, Vitamin E acetate, lemon juice concentrate, yellow dye #6, natural flavors, oleoresin turmeric, red dye #40, artificial flavors, blue dye #1

E. Granola
Health Food Store
Product name: Granola
Ingredients: Organic rolled oats, organic honey, organic safflower oil, organic sunflower seeds, organic whole wheat flour, organic spiced almonds, organic nonfat dry milk, organic sesame seeds, organic raisins
Supermarket
Product name: Kellogg's Granola
Ingredients: Whole oats, cold grain wheat, brown sugar, corn syrup, raisins, rice, sugar, almonds, partially hydrogenated cottonseed oil, glycerin, modified corn starch, salt, cinnamon, nonfat dry milk, high fructose corn syrup, polyglycerol esters of mono- and diglycerides, malt flavoring, alpha-tocopherol acetate, niacinamide, zinc oxide, sodium ascorbate, ascorbic acid, reduced iron, guar gum, BHT, cryodypyridoxine hydrochloride, riboflavin, Vitamin A palmitate, folic acid, thiamin hydrochloride, Vitamin D, Vitamin B

I hope the pattern here is obvious. The supermarket brand name options clearly contain many chemical ingredients that do not appear in the ingredients list of the equivalent health food store options. If you have the choice to eat something with ingredients you're familiar with, or something with a list of chemicals added to it, I hope you'll go with the ingredients you're familiar with because that product is going to be better for you.

I could do a hundred of these comparisons. There are huge and important differences between what's available in standard supermarkets and what's available in health food or whole food type stores. Keep in mind though, you must read the ingredients yourself. Just because it's in a health food store does not guarantee that it's good. Read the labels and follow my guidelines on what to avoid. When you purchase wisely, you'll be buying products that:

- ✔ Have few or no toxins
- ✔ Have more nutrition than their supermarket equivalent
- ✔ Taste better
- ✔ Make you feel better
- ✔ Will not give you gas, bloating, headaches, constipation, etc.
- ✔ Will not make you hungrier
- ✔ Will not make you fat
- ✔ Will not get you physically addicted
- ✔ And you'll be supporting small, independent, and in many cases local people who are trying to produce products that taste great and are good for you

When you go to your local supermarket and buy name brand products and/or products from major publicly traded food corporations, you're supporting the multinational companies that are hurting local growers and independent farmers, and causing massive amounts of illness and disease not only in America, but in countries around the world. It is my opinion that these large multinational corporations like Monsanto are exploiting and taking advantage of people through their clever use of advertising, and knowingly giving us food filled with chemicals that increase our appetite, get us physically addicted, and make us fat, all in the name of profit. Remember, I'm not being fanatical in advising you to eat more raw fruits, vegetables, nuts, and seeds. I'm recommending that you take small steps and go at a pace that's right for you.

Many of you may feel unwilling to drastically change your eating habits. For example, some of you love snack food and can't imagine giving up treats. That's fine. Go to the health food store and try different kinds of snacks to munch on. Many of them are incredibly delicious. As I write this, I'm thinking about some sweet snacks I recently purchased at my health food store. The first one has four ingredients and no chemicals: Pure raw carob, coconut, pure cane crystals, pure maple syrup. All of the ingredients are organic, raw, and real living food. They taste amazing. Another has these ingredients: Raw organic sunflower seeds, raw organic raisins, raw organic bananas, raw organic maple syrup, and fennel. This snack is sweet and tastes fantastic. Another one is an incredible almond brittle made with raw almonds, pure vanilla beans and crystals of pure cane. It's simple, real, and all natural. And here's the great part: Last night, to see how I would feel, I ate a huge bag of this almond brittle in one sitting. I didn't feel bloated, didn't get a sugar rush, my mood didn't go up or down—I felt absolutely fine and I slept like a baby. If I had done the same thing with some almond or peanut brittle made by a large, publicly traded corporation, I would have felt horrible, bloated, gassy and would have tossed and turned all night.

Just remember that name brand products and large multinational publicly traded corporations are investing tens of millions of dollars in research to find out what the hot buttons are to get you to buy their products. Don't believe their slick ads, and don't believe what's written on the front of the package. Read the ingredients. But do remember as you read them that *in addition* to the chemicals listed there, some of the toxins that were used to process the food may *not,* in fact, be listed. Yes, many toxins that are in the food *do not have to be listed on the ingredients.*

Here is an excerpt from the most recent guidelines of the FDA:

> **"Is it necessary to declare ingredients in "trace", i.e., incidental amounts? Can sulfites be considered incidental additives?**
>
> **Answer:** FDA does not define "trace amounts"; however, there are some exemptions for declaring ingredients present in "incidental" amounts in a finished food. If an ingredient is present at an incidental level and has no functional or technical effect in the finished product, then it need not be declared on the label."

There you have it. *"If an ingredient is present at an incidental level and has no functional or technical effect in the finished product, then it need not be declared on the label."* Do you see why this does not serve the public well? Who determines whether something has a "functional effect?" If the chemical has no functional effect, then why can't they omit it? And if they're going to include it, how can they know for sure that it will have no adverse effect on the people who consume it? The answer is *they can't know that for sure.* Monsanto is famous for getting away with this kind of thing. They put out harmful chemicals, like saccharine, for instance. Then they declare it "safe" with the FDA's approval, when it's anything *but* safe. It causes cancer; and only after whistle blowers prove the danger, do they make any change to what they're doing.

It's estimated that over 95 percent of all food products have as many as 300 added chemicals that are not listed on the label. This happens because companies have persuaded the FDA that the chemical "has no functional or technical effect on the product." This is the sad truth. This is power of the food industry. And this is why, if you want to eliminate and prevent sickness and disease, you need to stop buying food made by major corporations.

Restaurants

I'm often questioned about eating in restaurants. There are vast differences in the kinds of restaurants you may patronize. I'm not talking about the food. I'm talking about the kind of restaurant. Most restaurants have the following problems:

1. In order to make a profit they have to buy the cheapest food available. Restaurants get their food primarily from large, bulk food suppliers that supply hundreds of restaurants in a given area.

2. Much of the food you eat in any restaurant hasn't been cooked at the restaurant; rather, it's simply been finished off or heated up. This gets worse with restaurants that are vast in number, like fast food places or franchises.

3. Most restaurants use microwave ovens to reheat the food right before serving.

4. Most restaurants, like large food manufacturers, use frying oil all day and in some cases for days on end. The problem with this is once you heat the oil for frying it goes rancid quickly. All of the food that comes out of the rancid oil is carcinogenic.

Recently, I went to a nice restaurant and was about to order, but before doing so, I had some questions. I love fresh guacamole and often make it at home with fresh, raw, organic ingredients. It's absolutely delicious. Guacamole was on the menu so I asked if it was made fresh. The waiter told me that yes, it was. I inquired further. "So you actually take avocados and mash them up in the kitchen, or does it come in a prepackaged mix?" And he said, "Oh, well we do get a mix, but we add water and make it fresh every day."

His idea of fresh and my idea of fresh were completely different. This guacamole was *not* made in the back with fresh avocados, tomatoes, lime juice, onions, etc. Instead, it came as a powdered mix to which water was added. When I asked what the ingredients of the mix were, of course he didn't know. I persuaded him to go and find the package and bring me the ingredient list. There were over three dozen ingredients on the label, including monosodium glutamate.

I asked if the *salad* was fresh. He thought for a moment and said, "No. It actually comes in bags that have been prepackaged." The problem with this, of course, is that in order to retain freshness the "fresh salad" has to be sprayed with chemicals. I asked if the *chicken* was fresh, or did *it* come prepackaged, too. Not surprisingly, it came prepackaged and frozen. Virtually all of the sauces, all of the mixes, and all of the flavoring agents used came in boxes, cans, or packages. This is the unfortunate problem with a lot of restaurant food.

> Even making some simple modifications to your diet could have a dramatic impact.

So, what can you do? Basically, you can be a fanatic and not eat in any restaurant unless it's an all natural, totally organic one, or you can simply eat really well at home and stay away from chains, franchises, and fast food as best you can. When you go to a good quality restaurant, simply ask if you may tour the kitchen and see some of the food being prepared. Most managers welcome this. It'll give you a chance to meet the manager and/or the owner and inquire about how the different dishes are made. Then you can see which dish or dishes include the highest quality and the freshest ingredients. I ask a few questions and make some intelligent choices. Bear in mind, when it comes to eating out, you have to care, but not so much that it makes you crazy. Do what you feel comfortable with, and don't be stressed out about your decisions.

I have a close friend who's not only a vegetarian, but also only eats raw food. She's not stressed out or fanatical about it, that's just what she eats. We went to a restaurant and I ordered some salmon sushi. I knew the salmon was caught in the wild, and the brown rice was made with pure ingredients. I liked the cucumber and onion salad they made as well. The fresh ginger and wasabi were also delicious and made fresh at the restaurant. Although the restaurant does not use organic ingredients, it's a matter of degree. My meal could be classified as relatively healthy. Far from ideal, but also far from something you'd find in a fast food restaurant. At least there were no hydrogenated oils, monosodium glutamate, aspartame or massive amounts of chemicals. My friend, being a vegetarian and a raw foodist, had limited options, but her attitude about what she wanted was the key. She inquired about her choices and made her selections. We had lovely conversation, and her food was secondary in nature to our discussions. She wasn't stressed or uptight. She wasn't judgmental or pushing her ideas and values upon me. Maybe someday I'll eat raw food exclusively too. For right now, I love my organic lamb, chicken, beef and various kinds of cooked food. The point is, knowing all this information doesn't mean you have to do it *all* in order to receive benefits. Do a little or a lot, based on what you feel good about. Even making some simple modifications to your diet could have a dramatic impact.

CHAPTER 10

Still Not Convinced?

This book is filled with some very basic premises from which our conclusions are derived. The most basic is that there *are* natural, non-drug, and nonsurgical ways to prevent and cure virtually every disease. The FDA, the FTC, and the pharmaceutical industry work diligently to prevent you from learning about this information. The news media, including newspapers, magazines, television, and radio, are biased toward the pharmaceutical industry and present half-truths and outright lies in relation to healthcare. If you're still not persuaded that this is true consider these thought provoking ideas:

1. Still not convinced "it's all about the money"? Then consider this:

✔ The *Associated Press* has reported *"drug companies are seeing that cancer can be lucrative."* The article goes on to say how drug companies will be making billions of dollars in profits by selling cancer fighting drugs, even though they *do not work.* The article exposes the fact that curing cancer would be devastating to companies. Companies make money as long as people have cancer and they remain convinced that they need to take drugs. The article also exposes the fact that no research is being done by these drug companies on natural remedies for the treatment of cancer or on the *prevention* of cancer. The big money for these companies is making sure that more people get cancer and more people are brainwashed into buying their overpriced, ineffective and dangerous drugs.

✔ *USA Today* reported that biotech stock prices soared after cancer drug good news. The article pointed out the fact that publicly traded drug companies have only one goal: To increase profits, which means selling more drugs. The article never mentioned if the drugs were effective at preventing or curing cancer. It talked about how much money the companies would make by selling the drugs.

✔ Dozens of companies have been found guilty of failing to recall dangerous products. Several years ago Graco children's products agreed to pay a record $4 million penalty for hiding negative information about problems with their car seats, highchairs, strollers, and other products that resulted in hundreds of injuries and at least six deaths. This is an outrage. The corporate officers and directors should be held accountable for the murder of six people. These individuals made the decision to let people suffer and die so that they could make more money. This goes on all of the time in business. For every company that's caught there are hundreds of other violations that are not exposed. It's always *all about the money*.

✔ I was offered $50 million to recommend certain products when I wrote the first edition of the *Natural Cures* book. The individuals who made this offer even came up with a sophisticated plan of wiring money to numbered Swiss bank accounts. I can assure you that these types of bribes and payoffs are happening regularly in the news media, on television, radio, newspapers, and magazines. I've been offered positive stories on major news stations and in magazines and newspapers *if* I spend huge amounts of money in advertising. This type of corruption is rampant.

✔ Corporations do not want to provide good quality products. They want to get your money. One way to do this is to manufacture products that are of low quality and are guaranteed to break. This way, manufacturers can sell you outrageously priced extended service plans. Consider this when you buy an electronic device such as a computer. Sixty percent of all electronics break down in the first year. The profit made by retailers and the manufacturers in repairing and/or selling new equipment is astronomical. This is done purposely. Where's the Federal Trade Commission? The FTC is not protecting the consumers; it's protecting the profits of the large publicly traded corporations. Similarly, drug companies do not want to cure and prevent disease. They do not care about your health. They do not care about finding out why people are sick or discovering the best ways to prevent sickness and cure illness. Drug companies only want to develop and *sell* patented drugs. This is evidenced by the fact that the majority of their money is not spent on verifying that their drugs are effective and/or safe. The majority of their money is spent on marketing to convince you that you need drugs and that you must buy drugs.

✔ Newspapers, magazines, television, and radio commonly bad mouth all natural products, while at the same time run ads for products that they are *not* bashing. This is done purposely. It occurs blatantly on web sites. It's important to note that there are almost never reports done on companies or products that are the sponsors of those TV stations, radio stations, newspapers, magazines, or web sites. Consider that when companies provide advertising revenue to a "news organization" you never see them run negative stories about those products or companies. Why? Because they don't want to bite the hand that feeds them. But this is an inherent limitation and one that does a disservice to the public. If a company wants to avoid bad press, they can simply payoff the news outlets with advertising money.

✔ Health food and vitamin companies are being gobbled up by the pharmaceutical industry either owned directly or indirectly by them. This is so the drug companies can control all natural vitamins and minerals. When the pharmaceutical companies control this industry, they will either raise the prices dramatically and begin charging much more for all natural herbs, vitamins, and minerals, or they will simply take them off the market,therefore making it impossible for you to have natural options to drugs. This is being done systematically so that the pharmaceutical industry can control and monopolize healthcare. This should be a violation of antitrust laws. The politicians do nothing. The FTC, the agency entrusted with protecting consumers against antitrust violations and monopolies such as this, does nothing. This is corruption at the highest levels of government.

✔ Many "newsletters" or books promote certain supplements. Most people do not know that the owners of these newsletters or books are the same people who actually sell the supplements. This is misleading and fraudulent, but very profitable for the big corporations. Magazines and newspapers commonly run positive articles on products if those companies commit to large advertising contracts. What this means is that you can't believe much of what you read in magazines and newspapers, because you don't know if the article is really a payoff for the prodigious amount of advertising the publisher receives.

2. Still not convinced that the FTC and FDA, as well as maybe TV, radio, and news organizations, are suppressing and censoring information? Then consider this:

✔ The natural supplement ephedra was banned, but the pharmaceutical version, ephedrine, was not banned. The natural version was taken off the market, but the dangerous chemically produced synthetic version is still allowed to be sold. This shows how the FDA protects the pharmaceutical industry.

✔ Drug advertising is everywhere. You see drug ads on TV, hear them on radio, and read them in newspapers and in magazines. Drug companies sponsor sporting events and fill our mailboxes with direct mail campaigns promoting their drugs. These drug ads in many cases have been deemed misleading and/or false, yet the FTC has taken no action against any pharmaceutical company for producing false and misleading ads even though these promotional materials are encouraging people under false pretenses to use these dangerous and ineffective drugs. There has never been a drug ad rejected by a television or radio station, newspaper, or magazine. However television stations, newspapers, magazines, and radio stations will routinely reject advertising for all natural herbal products, homeopathic products, vitamins, minerals, or books that are critical of the pharmaceutical industry.

✔ The most obvious example that the government, as well as the news organizations are suppressing and censoring information is the Monsanto exposé that was squashed by Fox. This is the story where two journalists did a report exposing the growth hormone that Monsanto manufactures and how it was being injected into dairy cows, potentially causing illness and disease and tainting the milk with poisons that harm humans as well. This true story was squashed by Fox. Why? To protect the profits of Monsanto.

3. Still not convinced that the media is biased, deceiving, and lying to you about many topics? Then consider this:

✔ Have you ever read a bad article written about a news organization's sponsors? You'd be hard pressed to recall one of those. It just doesn't happen. This is a blatant example of how the media is biased and succumbs to the whims and pressures of its sponsors. The news media is the mouthpiece of the large corporations that buy the advertising. The *majority* of advertising is from the pharmaceutical industry and the food industry; therefore, it is virtually impossible to hear the truth about how the food being produced by large publicly traded corporations is in fact giving us disease and making us fat, and how the drugs are ineffective and giving us disease.

✔ Many news articles are written by individuals who are on the payroll of the companies profiled in those articles. An example a few years back was an article with the headline: "Despite Known Hazards, Many Potentially Dangerous Dietary Supplements Continue to be Used." This article was written by a doctor who was on the payroll of a drug company. The story wasn't "news." It wasn't true, nor was it unbiased journalism. It was a debunking campaign by the pharmaceutical industry to turn people away from safe and effective natural remedies, and instead, to continue to brainwash people into believing drugs are the only answer for illness and disease. This continues to happen.

✔ Pharmaceutical companies set up and pay for web sites by the hundreds debunking natural remedies. Usually, a small group of people actually runs and maintains hundreds of web sites, so an individual consumer thinks that there are multiple independent organizations around the world saying how bad natural remedies are and how good drugs are. This is propaganda in its most flagrant form.

✔ The four basic food group model promoted for years was actually invented by, promoted by, and funded by the dairy association. The food pyramid today was put into effect by our government after massive lobbying by the food industry. The four basic food groups and the food pyramid have nothing to do with health and nutrition, but are designed to brainwash people into eating a certain way for the benefit of the food industry.

✔ The media hides the truth about the dangers of nonprescription and prescription drugs. There are very few articles written about how lethal over-the-counter nonprescription and prescription drugs really are. However, the number of articles that have been written broadcasting the dangers of natural supplements such as herbs, vitamins and minerals is staggering. The fact is drugs, both over-the-counter nonprescription and prescription ones, are infinitely more dangerous than any vitamin, mineral or herb. There are virtually no reported cases of anyone dying from taking a natural supplement in its proper dose. However, there are hundreds of thousands of documented deaths that have occurred by taking an over-the-counter nonprescription or prescription drug in its proper dosage.

✔ Whistleblowers now report that all forms of media, including radio, TV, newspapers, and magazines, are in fact owned by the sponsors. There are secret meetings with the sponsors who dictate the content of all programming and topics covered or not covered in the media outlets.

4. Still not convinced that right now your body is loaded with toxins causing you all types of illness, disease, depression, stress, and anxiety? Then consider this:

✔ All injections from Botox, collagen, insulin and vaccines are loaded with poisonous toxins. Many of these are animal based and are filled with deadly pathogens and chemicals.

✔ There are so many toxins in our environment and food that even people who live in the most remote parts of the world have been found to have toxins in their fat cells. And this is the case even though the toxins do not exist in their local environment. This is a toxic world, and no one is immune. You are filled with toxins right now.

✔ A study showed that traces of industrial strength fire retardant have turned up in wild and farm-raised salmon around the world. Farm-raised salmon has been found to have troubling levels of PCBs, a known cancer causing agent. When you eat this food the toxins go inside *you*.

✔ The newspaper *The Daily Mail* reported, "Ready to eat salad linked with birth defects… Cancer hazard is in packed salad." The article goes on to expose how premixed ready to eat salad is washed with chlorine. The chlorine is bad enough, but it combines with chemicals naturally present in lettuce to create chlorine byproducts, which can be even more hazardous to your health.

✔ The government has found traces of rocket fuel chemical in milk, green leaf lettuce, and drinking water. The government also acknowledges that these chemicals adversely affect the thyroid, which potentially can make you fat and lead to dozens of other diseases.

✔ *Reuters* reported that air pollution is so bad that it is adversely affecting lung function in teenagers.

✔ *The Daily News* newspaper reported that certain cookies are having hydrogenated oil removed since there is overwhelming evidence that these trans fats cause obesity, clogging of the arteries, heart disease, strokes, and death. This is significant because you have been eating massive amounts of trans fats for the last thirty years, which is one of the major reasons sickness and disease are at an all-time high.

✔ *Reuters* reported that mercury is being released from coal fired power plants and is one of the contributing causes of an increase in autism and other health disorders. It is also believed that whether you live near a power plant or not, you are still affected since once mercury is in the atmosphere it circulates around the globe.

✔ It has been reported that the feed used in U.S. cattle production may be routinely tainted with poisons and disease. The rules and regulations relating to feed are not being complied with. Cattle producers are more interested in making money than safety. They routinely break the law by not complying with safety standards. This means the beef that we're eating is loaded with toxins, poisons, and disease-causing chemicals.

✔ *USA Today* reported the air pollution from other countries drifts into the United States. We breathe in more toxins today than ever before in history. These toxins stay in our body and cause disease.

✔ William Campbell, M.D., stated, "Your daily shower could be killing you softly with the same toxins used to kill lab rats and [used] in chemical weapons." The toxic substances in most municipal water systems have been used in the past to kill laboratory animals and as a weapon of war. It may be more dangerous to shower in municipal water than to drink it.

✔ Genetically modified food is rampant in our food supply. It does not have to be labeled as genetically altered. Now, food manufacturers in a quest to make more money, are changing the nature of things by genetically manufacturing animals and fish. Though genetically modified salmon hasn't been approved by the U.S. yet, just recently in Canada the American company AquaBounty received the green light to manufacture modified fish eggs. Eating genetically modified food means we are ingesting more poisons and toxins.

5. Still not convinced that politicians and various government agencies are corrupt, out of control, and operating un-policed? Then consider this:

✔ The government has changed the definitions of some of the most basic things we know. Example: There was a reported list of the healthiest states in America. Health, in this particular survey, was defined as the number of hospital beds per 1,000 people, and the percentage of children who got all of their recommended vaccinations. They were defining healthiest states as those where people were getting the greatest number of drugs and the most surgery. How insane. The definition for "spices" now includes thousands of deadly chemicals. Roast beef doesn't have to be real roast beef anymore, it can be a man-made product and still be called "roast beef."

✔ Did you know that if you have a child who's been diagnosed with cancer, not giving that child chemotherapy and other drugs can be a criminal offense?

✔ Political insiders are now blowing the whistle on how politics works. Report after report show that politicians have little interest in what's best for the country, the communities, or individual citizens. Every politician has simple objectives:

(a) to get re-elected, (b) to increase their political power and influence, and (c) to increase their personal wealth.

✔ In the last several decades there have been dozens of politicians' "suicides" and accidental deaths; however, none reported as "murders." Doesn't it make you think or at least suspect foul play and corruption?

6. Still not convinced that the FDA is working with big business and major drug companies allowing them to deceive the public and flood the public marketplace with dangerous products? Then consider this:

✔ Cigarettes are obviously bad; however, they are the only product in America where the ingredients do not have to be listed. How can this be? Well, consider that the FDA is in charge and that the politicians who receive huge amounts of donations and lobbying by the tobacco industry tell the FDA what to do.

✔ Federal law prohibits the FDA from using experts with financial conflicts of interest, but the FDA has waived the restriction close to 1,000 times since 1998. Although the FDA does not reveal when financial conflicts exist, since 1992 it has kept the details of any conflict secret so it is not possible to determine the amount of money or the drug companies involved. Two articles ran in *Reuters News* and *USA Today* reporting that 54 percent of the experts the FDA asked for advice on which medicines should be approved for sale have a direct financial interest in the drugs or topics they are evaluating. These financial conflicts of interest typically include stock ownership, consulting fees, or research grants. The *USA Today* article stated, "These pharmaceutical experts, about 300 on eighteen different advisory committees, make decisions that affect the health of millions of Americans and billions of dollars in drug sales. With few exceptions, the FDA follows the committee's advice." The scary part is these people who are making these decisions have a direct financial interest and they benefit based on the decisions they make. The article concluded that at 92 percent of the meetings, at least one member had a financial conflict of interest. At 55 percent of the meetings, half or more of the FDA advisors had conflicts of interest. Conflicts were most frequent at the fifty-seven meetings where broader issues were discussed; 92 percent of those members had conflicts. At the 102 meetings dealing with the fate of a specific drug,33 percent of the experts had a direct financial interest.

✔ The pharmaceutical industry has more influence with the FDA than the public realizes. In an edition of the prestigious medical journal *Lancet*, editor Richard Horton claimed that the FDA has become a servant to the drug industry. An example: Even though there are multiple deaths caused by certain drugs, the FDA does not recall them from the market, but suggests adding a warning. The *Los Angeles Times* reported that the FDA has withheld safety information from labels that physicians say would call into question the use of the drugs. In the last twenty years, over a million people were killed by drugs that were approved, but never should have been. Before 1990, 60 percent of drugs submitted to the FDA were approved. Today over 80 percent are approved. The *Los Angeles Times* reported that seven killer drugs that were approved by the FDA, and yet were so deadly that they had to be withdrawn, generated over $5 billion for the pharmaceutical industry before the recall. Most shocking is that the FDA knowingly puts children at risk. According to the *LA Times* article, the agency never warned doctors not to administer a drug to infants or other children, even though eight youngsters who were given this drug in clinical studies died. Pediatricians prescribed it widely for infants afflicted with gastric reflux, a common digestive disorder. Patients and their doctors had no way of knowing that the FDA, in August 1996, had found the drug to be "not approvable for children." "We never knew that," said the father of a three-month old son who died on October 28, 1997, after taking the drug. "To me, that means they took my kid as a guinea pig to see if it would work." By the time the drug was pulled, the FDA had received reports of twenty-four deaths of children under age six who had been given this drug. By then, the drug had generated U.S. sales of over $2.5 billion for the drug company.

✔ An FDA insider said, "People are aware that turning down a drug for approval is going to cause problems with officials higher up in the FDA. Before I came to the FDA, I always assumed things were done properly. I've now lost faith in taking any prescription medication."

✔ According to one *Los Angeles Times* story, seven drugs approved by the FDA were later found to be ineffective and fatal. How the FDA approved these drugs is still a mystery. They obviously relied on misleading and/or false studies. Keep in mind all studies submitted to the FDA are always paid for and produced by the drug company that's seeking approval. These drugs were not needed. They weren't miracle drugs created to save lives. They were simply drugs designed to increase profits of the drug companies. One was for heartburn. Another was a diet pill, and a third was a painkiller. Six of the drugs were never proved to offer any lifesaving benefits and the seventh, an antibiotic, was ultimately deemed totally unnecessary because there were other antibiotics available that had already proven to be safer than this deadly antibiotic. These drugs did not have to be approved, but they were pushed for approval so that the drug companies could market them and make billions of dollars. These seven drugs had to be pulled off the market. The FDA repeatedly allows dangerous drugs to be approved and sold because of the pressure put on it by the drug industry.

✔ According to the *Los Angeles Times*, back in 1988, only 4 percent of new drugs introduced into the world market were approved first by the FDA. Ten years later in 1998, the FDA's first in the world approval spiked to 66 percent. It appears that the easiest agency in the world to approve a new drug, regardless of the safety, has become the FDA. The FDA was once the world's leading organization when it came to the safety of drugs it approved. Now the FDA seems to be more interested in the sales and profits of the drug companies than the safety of consumers.

✔ One particular drug the FDA approved and deemed "safe and effective" was pulled within the first year because it was linked to five deaths, as well as to the removal of many of the patients' colons and other major bowel surgeries. Other drugs called "safe and effective" by the FDA were later proven to cause heart valve damage, liver damage, pancreas damage, prostate cancer, colon cancer, impotency, infertility, heart attack, and stroke.

✔ The *Los Angeles Times* reported that, seven specific drugs that were called "safe and effective" resulted in a minimum of a thousand reported deaths. Other experts say that number is much higher, and could be as high as twenty-thousand deaths. All from drugs the FDA called "safe and effective." What isn't recorded are the potential hundreds of thousands of patients who took these drugs that developed other severe medical conditions such as liver damage, heart problems, cancer, diabetes, digestive issues, etc. The most outrageous thing is that all of these new medical conditions will be treated by the medical doctors with surgeries and/or more drugs. The needless pain and suffering of hundreds of thousands of people, and the deaths of countless more, is being ignored, all in the name of profit.

✔ The *Los Angeles Times* on Tuesday, April 6, 2004, quoted Harvard psychiatrist Dr. Joseph Glen Mullen: "Evidence that the FDA is suppressing a report linking suicide to drugs is an outrage given the public health and safety issues at stake." The FDA has information that antidepressants caused children to be twice as likely to show suicidal behavior. The article shows how the FDA claims that there is no conclusive scientific evidence linking antidepressants and potential suicide behavior. However, the article goes on to say that there is absolute evidence that the FDA is suppressing and hiding the information so that the drug companies can continue to sell drugs.

✔ Nonfatal skin cancers are the number one cancer. The four other most common kinds are breast, prostate, lung, and colorectal, which is cancer of the colon. Research and observations strongly suggest that the people most prone to getting these cancers are those who have taken the most nonprescription and prescription drugs and who have eaten the most fast food, yet the FDA does nothing to inform the public of the dangers of these two activities.

✔ In 2006, the *New York Times* reported that a study found Johnson & Johnson's popular treatment for congestive heart failure, Natrecor, caused reduced kidney function. In 2010, the *Los Angeles Times* reported that a subsequent study dismissed the links to kidney problems, but found that drug was "not effective."

✔ Experts say the drug Zoloft causes dementia.

✔ The *Associated Press* reported that drugs used to treat prostate cancer make men prone to broken bones.

✔ The FDA effectively silenced one of its own drug experts who exposed the safety concerns about the profitable drug Vioxx. This is proof that the FDA is more interested in protecting the profits of the drug companies than the safety of consumers.

✔ A previously unpublished internal survey of FDA scientists points to potentially dangerous gaps in the approval and marketing of prescription drugs. The internal secret survey showed that the FDA does not adequately monitor the safety of prescription drugs once they are on the market, and the majority of FDA scientists do not believe that the labeling decisions adequately address key safety concerns. It also showed that an alarming percentage of FDA scientists themselves were not confident that the final decisions adequately addressed the safety of drugs. The most alarming piece of information to come out of this secret internal survey was the number of scientists that said they have been pressured to approve or recommend drugs despite their own reservations about safety, efficacy, or quality of the drug. This means that the senior executives at the FDA are more interested in protecting the profits of the drug companies than they are about the safety of the consumer.

✔ In 2005 the *Wall Street Journal* reported that too many unproven drugs were getting approved by the FDA.

✔ In 2005, in the wake of the Vioxx scandal, the *Chicago Tribune* reported that the FDA was caught in the middle of a "drug safety conflict." The article suggested that the drug industry actually controls what is happening at the FDA.

✔ The FDA reviewed the drug Celebrex. The FDA's advisory panel recommended that Celebrex stay on the market. The amazing thing is that the members of this advisory panel are all in effect on the payroll of the drug company that sells Celebrex! Can someone stand up, and yell *conflict of interest* please?

✔ The FDA has admitted that two eczema creams cause cancer.

✔ The *Wall Street Journal* reported that cholesterol lowering drugs fail to benefit patients. Cholesterol drugs are the number one selling drugs in the world. They make the most profits for the drug industry, but the fact is cholesterol reducing drugs do not do anything to reduce the potential dangers of heart disease. A study showed that there were no heart health benefits after four months and no significant benefits after two years. However, the study did show that continued use of these cholesterol lowering drugs caused illness and disease.

✔ The *Associated Press* reported that consumer groups blasted the new cholesterol guidelines. Most of the heart disease experts who urged more people to take cholesterol lowering drugs have been exposed to have made huge amounts of money from the companies selling those medicines. "It's outrageous they didn't provide disclosure of the conflicts of interest," said Merrill Goozner with the Center for Science in the Public Interest. Folks, this happens all of the time. Remember, too, that most studies for new and existing drugs are paid for and funded by their own manufacturers.

✔ The New York attorney general sued the pharmaceutical giant Glaxo/Smith/Kline saying it committed fraud by withholding information about the dangers of its antidepressant drugs to children. This should not be the only suit filed. It is important you know that every major pharmaceutical company withholds information about the ineffectiveness and dangers of their drugs. It is important you know that the drug companies and the FDA know that the drugs do not work and are actually dangerous and cause disease, yet they're hiding and withholding this information from the public.

✔ The *Associated Press* reported that the drug Avastin increases the risk of heart ailments including chest pain, strokes, mini-strokes, and heart attacks. This means that this drug can kill the people who take it. (It's interesting to note that every article I am reporting on here that talks about drugs also has a heavy emphasis on the stock price and how this news is affecting shareholder value. I cannot emphasize enough that drug companies are *publicly traded companies* whose only objective is to make profit. They do not want to cure or prevent disease.)

✔ *USA Today* reported that a grieving father, Liam Grant, spent a $1 million nest egg to investigate the drug Accutane. He believed that this drug caused his son to commit suicide. Allegedly, Liam was offered hundreds of thousands of dollars to drop the case. After multiple lawsuits Roche Pharmaceuticals stopped selling the drug in 2009. Accutane is no longer available, however its generic version is still available outside of the U.S.

✔ Whistleblowers have reported that internal documents at both the drug manufacturers and FDA show that drugs, both prescription and nonprescription, have no positive effects in over 70 percent of the people who use them. However, these same documents show that all nonprescription and prescription drugs have negative side effects in 100 percent of the people who use them.

7. Still not convinced that the pharmaceutical industry pushes drug sales and usage at all costs, and has an insatiable desire for increasing profits? Then consider this:

✔ Schools get money each month for every child they have on a psychiatric drug, including Ritalin or Adderall. This gives a major incentive for schools to get and keep kids on drugs.

✔ Doctors routinely get visits from pharmaceutical sales reps. These sales reps do not tell doctors how to cure and prevent disease. These sales people have sophisticated presentations designed to tell doctors how they can make more money by prescribing more drugs. These presentations have almost zero information on the safety or effectiveness of these drugs. The concern is not the patient; the emphasis is on how doctors can make more money.

✔ Doctors on government advisory panels make recommendations for drugs while being paid huge sums of money by the manufacturers of those same drugs.

✔ Drug companies routinely sponsor foundations' research. For example, Amgen gave $150,000 for research done by the Kidney Foundation. Remember, all foundations, all charities, and all research conducted on drugs is almost always paid for by the drug companies themselves, which therefore guarantees the results they want.

8. Still not convinced that all over-the-counter nonprescription and prescription drugs are poisons, causing you physical and emotional harm? Then consider this:

✔ Depending on who you listen to, either the third or fourth leading cause of death in America are doctors. This is because doctors routinely prescribe drugs that kill their patients, or perform surgeries that are unsuccessful. Either the patients die, or the doctors misdiagnose the illness and do the wrong thing which causes the person to die.

✔ In 2013, the *Journal of Patient Safety* said that "between 210,000-440,000 die each year" because of mistakes made in hospitals. "Things like unnecessary surgery, medical errors, negative effects of drugs, etc., cause almost as many deaths as heart disease and cancer." This figure does not include people who are permanently maimed, injured, or develop serious other medical conditions due to drugs and surgical procedures.

✔ Lowering cholesterol will not prevent a heart attack.

✔ An aspirin a day can give you gastrointestinal bleeding.

✔ It's been reported that over seven million Americans above sixty-five receive prescriptions for drugs that a panel of experts deemed inappropriate for use by the elderly because of potentially dangerous side effects.

✔ According to a study in the *Journal of the American Medical Association*, every prescription drug has dangerous side effects, and over 20 percent of these drugs come on the market without any warnings.

9. Still not convinced that aspartame (NutraSweet®) is one of the most dangerous food additives available today? Then consider this:

✔ NutraSweet® (aspartame) contains methanol, a wood alcohol which is a deadly poison. Aspartame was approved based on 112 studies submitted to the FDA by the original manufacturer, G.D. Searle, which was acquired by Monsanto. All of these studies were paid for and funded by the drug company. Critics who look at these studies, most notably the fifteen pivotal studies that the FDA based its approval on, are astonished that anyone could deduce that aspartame is safe. It's amazing that one of the subjects in the study died within a year after taking aspartame. Some of the studies showed people who were taking aspartame were having brain seizures. Once the aspartame was withdrawn from the subjects' diets, the brain seizures stopped. All of the studies were brief, (just a few months) and consisted of few subjects. The FDA has received more complaints from people who've consumed aspartame and who've had more major negative side effects than any other approved food, yet no action has ever been taken by the agency. In 2003, a former investigator for the FDA exposed aspartame as a toxin that never should have been approved. In 2013, the dairy industry began petitioning the FDA to allow aspartame in milk.

10. Still not convinced that your thoughts and energy are important to your health, and can have a major impact on physiology? Then consider this:

✔ In testing people diagnosed with multiple personality disorder, thought has been shown to do what is otherwise believed to be scientifically impossible. In one case, a person's blood was tested and found to be free of diabetes. Within minutes, when his personality changed, the blood was taken again and the person was tested positive for diabetes. This is physically impossible according to scientists, but the tests confirmed it nonetheless. This shows that the mind can do things to the body, even change body chemistry.

✔ An experiment was conducted to determine if thoughts can affect DNA. DNA was placed in a container; it was discovered that the DNA changed its shape according to the feelings, thoughts, and emotions of the researchers. When the researchers felt gratitude, love, and appreciation, the DNA responded by relaxing and the strands unwound; the length of the DNA extended. When the researchers felt anger, fear, frustration, or stress, the DNA responded by tightening up; it became shorter and switched off many of its codes. This could be why people feel shut down when they experience stress and negative emotions. The DNA codes were reversed and switched back on when feelings of love, joy, gratitude, and appreciation were felt by the researchers. This experiment was later followed up by testing HIV-positive patients. It turned out there was a three hundred times increase in resistance to viruses and bacteria when the HIV-positive patients felt love, gratitude, and appreciation. The bottom line is thoughts, feelings, emotions, and "energy" have a positive or negative effect on your DNA structure and can give you disease or cure you of disease.

✔ Ann Harrington, a professor of science at Harvard University wrote an article for *Spirituality and Health* magazine entitled "Miracle Cures—Tapping the Power of Make Believe Medicine." In it, Harrington showed that a placebo actually "cures" disease. She goes on to point out that in reality, the placebo does nothing except help the person believe that his or her disease will be cured and it's the patient's own mind and belief that cures the disease. To demonstrate this, the article gives examples where placebos are moderately effective when given as a little white tablet, but *more* effective when given as a big red capsule, and effective nearly100 percent of the time when the patient has to roll up his or her sleeve and get an injection. In effect, as the belief level increases the power of the mind increases as well and the body heals itself.

✔ In the book *The Hidden Messages in Water*, by Masaru Emoto, it is explained that the structure of water is dramatically affected by thoughts. Candice Pert, Ph.D. says that thought alone can completely change the body. This book shows the pictures so you can see how dramatically the water is changed structurally simply by thoughts.

✔ In research, when a person begins to worry and have stress, the body's pH can go from alkaline to acidic in a matter of minutes. Thoughts can bring on disease faster than any other cause.

11. Still not convinced that organic food is much better for you? Then consider this:

✔ A February 2003 study published in the *Journal of Agriculture and Food Industry* showed organically grown berries contain up to 58 percent more antioxidants than those grown conventionally.

✔ A 1993 study published in the *Journal of Applied Nutrition* showed that over the course of two years organic foods contained up to four times as many trace minerals, thirteen times more selenium and twenty times more calcium and magnesium than commercially grown produce, and also had significantly fewer heavy metals, including 25 percent less lead and 40 percent less aluminum.

12. Still not convinced that we are losing the war on cancer and cancer is getting worse every year? Then consider this:

✔ Every year, over 1.5 million Americans are diagnosed with cancer and the number is increasing. The probability that you will develop cancer is one in every two men and one in every three women, and it's getting worse. The war on cancer has been a total failure. Some scientists estimate that up to 70 percent of all cancers could be prevented simply by dietary change. The only legal remedies for cancer treatment are surgery, chemotherapy, and radiation. You can go to prison if you treat cancer with all natural methods even though they are more effective than surgery, chemotherapy and radiation, and have absolutely no negative side effects.

13. Still not convinced that the FDA suppresses information on natural cures? Then consider this:

✔ The *California Western Law Review* published an article entitled "Why Does the FDA Deny Access to Alternative Cancer Treatments?"

✔ Canadian scientist, Gaston Naessens, created an herbal blend called 714-X. This blend, as of 1991, has cured more than 1,000 people of cancer, as well as several AIDS patients. The FDA has attacked him.

✔ Jason Winters authored the book *Killing Cancer,* which has sold more than a million copies, about how he cured his cancer with herbs. He is quoted as saying, "I must tell you that I was scared about publishing a book talking about how herbs can cure cancer. I was not prepared to take on the billion dollar drug companies, the medical associations and doctors, all of whom would chew up and spit out anyone that would dare to say that possibly, just possibly, herbs can help." Winters outlines the typical fate of natural cancer cures and other cures that are advertised in U.S. publications. Usually the publication gets into a lot of trouble for printing it in the first place, and then all future publicity is stopped. The people selling the products are usually tricked into a phony suit about "practicing medicine without a license," or "selling drugs without a license," or " selling unregistered drugs." If the government can't stop them that way, they usually use another federal agency—the IRS, to attack them with some phony, trumped up income tax charge. Those who practice natural medicine, or sell natural remedies, live with the knowledge that they could be closed down any day.

✔ Virtually all violent acts committed by children in schools over the last ten years were committed by individuals who had been on prescribed psychiatric drugs, including the case in 2012 of the Newtown shooter, Adam Lanza who killed twenty-six people, twenty of them young children. This point was raised quickly after the Newtown event, and then quickly dropped by the mainstream media because (as we've explained) the news outlets are sponsored with advertising from the very drug companies that make these psychiatric drugs. These drugs increase the likelihood of suicide and dramatically increase the propensity for violent acts.

✔ Most drugs are physically addictive. Particularly pain medication, as evidenced by many celebrities who've been given medication by their doctor not knowing the addictive nature of the drugs.

14. Still not convinced that household cleaners are dangerous to your health? Then consider this:

✔ The *Associated Press* reported that deaths show dangers of household chemicals. This article explained how ALL household cleaners are chemicals that are highly toxic. They all can be fatal if they get into your system. They can be absorbed through the skin, through the fumes that you inhale, and of course, by accidentally drinking. Most people won't die immediately by inhaling the fumes, but the article points out that several people *have* died immediately as a result of mixing multiple cleaners together, which created deadly toxic fumes. If these chemicals in high concentrations can cause instantaneous death, then using these chemicals regularly and frequently obviously causes health problems. Exposure to them suppresses the immune system and leads to disease.

15. Still not convinced that the food produced by publicly traded companies and fast food restaurants is giving us disease and making us fat? Then consider this:

- ✔ *Reuters* reported that McDonald's has agreed to pay $8.5 million to settle a lawsuit because they were putting trans fats in their cooking oil. The lawsuit was filed by an activist seeking to raise awareness about the health dangers of trans fats in hydrogenated or partially hydrogenated oils. In 2008, McDonald's switched to a trans fat-free oil. However trans fats were just ONE of the many toxins in fast food and it took activism to change that. These companies will not change their destructive ways by their own volition.

- ✔ Kraft Foods was sued for knowingly putting dangerous trans fats in its food, most notably Oreos.

- ✔ An investigator for an animal rights group captured video showing chickens being kicked, stomped, and thrown against the wall by workers at a supplier for Kentucky Fried Chicken.

- ✔ Beef used for hamburger patties at fast food restaurants now contains enormous numbers of cattle that are being herded, fattened, slaughtered, and ground up together. This means meat from a single cow is not used in the hamburger patty; they are pooling bacteria from as many as a thousand different animals.

- ✔ The magazine *The Ecologist* points out that cosmetically perfect, irresistibly firm, brilliantly colored fruits and vegetables (like those in major supermarkets) taste like nothing because they're genetically modified and contain so many toxins.

- ✔ Samples of nonorganic chicken breasts (like those sold in major supermarkets) were found to be just 54 percent chicken. The rest was essentially fillers, i.e. toxins.

16. Still not convinced that natural remedies cure disease better than drugs, with no side effects? Then consider this:

- ✔ Licensed healthcare practitioners who use natural remedies instead of drugs and surgery report higher success rates than medical doctors using drugs and surgery. They also report virtually no negative side effects from treatments compared to medical doctors, who report negative side effects from treatments in virtually 100 percent of their patients.

- ✔ The *Associated Press* reported that walking may ward off Alzheimer's disease.

- ✔ *Reuters* reported that eating organic is shown to prevent and cure a host of various diseases.

- ✔ *Reuters* reported that the herbal remedy St. John's Wort is as effective, or more effective, in treating depression than drugs.

- ✔ The FDA finally admitted that extra virgin olive oil reduces the chances of coronary heart disease.

- ✔ *BBC* news reported that eating apples wards off colon cancer, and that apples prevent and can potentially cure cancer.

- ✔ The *Associated Press* reported that walking keeps weight in check.

- ✔ *ABC News* reported that relaxation techniques lower blood pressure.

- ✔ *Yahoo News* reported that herbs help ease children's illnesses, such as colds, skin allergies, and sleep problems. It also reported that the herbs worked more efficiently than drugs and had no side effects.

- ✔ Multiple studies have identified green tea as an anticancer agent.

- ✔ There is increased scientific validation for how homeopathy prevents and cures disease.

✔ Mangosteen juice, in studies, has been shown to prevent hardening of the arteries, protect the heart muscle, be beneficial in the treatment of Parkinson's disease, Alzheimer's disease and other forms of dementia, elevate mood and act as an antidepressant, prevent and arrest fungus, prevent bacterial infections, fight viruses, prevent gum disease, lower fever, prevent glaucoma and cataracts, increase energy and fight fatigue, promote anti-aging and weight loss, lower blood fat, have anti-tumor benefits, prevent cancer, lower blood pressure, lower blood sugar, and improve digestion.

17. Still not convinced that electromagnetic energy causes disease? Then consider this:

✔ College researchers believe electric light changes hormone levels in women and makes breast cancer more prevalent. The theory is that exposure to artificial, mostly florescent light, causes cellular damage that can lead to cancer, as well as dozens of other diseases.

✔ A Swedish study showed that people who hold cell phones to their head increase their risk of developing brain tumors. In the last few years evidence has been mounting to corroborate this study. In 2011, the World Health Organization issued a statement reversing its previous claim that no adverse health effects had been established. In its retraction, WHO said: "personal exposure IS possibly carcinogenic to humans."

✔ The cell phone industry has been just as harmful to public health as big tobacco. The similarities are eerily obvious. The cell phone industry was determined to deny any suggestion that its products might be dangerous even though years of negative research proved otherwise. One study showed that mobile phones emanate radio waves that damage the cells in the body, as well as DNA. Most shocking was the fact that the damage extended to the next generation of cells as well. The Cellular Telecommunications & Internet Association headed up a $28 million research program looking into the possible health effects from cellular phone use. Amazingly, the industry's own research showed that heavy cell phone users experience an increased rate of brain cancer deaths, development of tumors, genetic damage in the cells, as well as other negative health issues.

My most recent personal experience of how health care is a monopoly for the pharmaceutical industry was when I requested to take some blood tests. After walking in to a lab and asking for blood work to be performed, I was told it was against the law to do blood work without a prescription. It was appalling to me how the lawmakers created this monopoly for medical doctors. Reluctantly, I acquired a prescription. When I had the blood drawn and paid the bill, I asked when I could have my results. I was told it was against the law for them to release my test results to me. The results must be sent to a medical doctor. This was *my* blood, and *I* paid for the tests with *my* money, yet the law denies me direct access to the results. This is a good example of how lawmakers guarantee profits for medical doctors.

> I was told it was against the law for them to release my test results to me. The results must be sent to a medical doctor.

I could go on and on proving the many points referenced in this chapter and others. The evidence is overwhelming. Volumes of documentation, substantiation, and reports back up everything I say. Can you see why I'm mad as hell and not going to take it anymore?!

CHAPTER 11

Natural Cures for Specific Diseases

Stop! If you just bought this book and flipped to this chapter trying to find the "magic cure" for your specific disease, *please go back and start reading from the beginning.* Many important things are covered earlier and it's essential for you to understand and implement those things before you're ready for this chapter. If you start here you will not *get it.* You must understand how the medical system works and how you've been brainwashed. You must understand the cause of disease and the basic ways to cure yourself and bring your body to a state of balance where disease cannot exist. This chapter is designed *only* to give you suggestions for non-drug, nonsurgical things you can do to potentially address the symptoms that you may have.

If you're experiencing symptoms, the first question to ask is "What is *causing* them?" What most people ask is, "What can I do to *eliminate* the symptoms?" This is jumping the gun. First find out what's causing the symptoms, and then you can address the root cause by making changes. When you do this the symptoms vanish.

As I've mentioned before, the problem with standard drugs and surgery is that they only address the symptoms, they don't address the cause. This is a good modus operandi for the drug manufacturers; it makes them lots of money, but it's bad for you because it doesn't require that you change what created your illness (and the symptoms that come with it), so you're bound to get sick again. Eliminate the *cause* and the illness can't return, because the conditions that led to its creation no longer exist.

If someone approached you and said, "Every time I hit my foot with a hammer it hurts. How do I stop the pain?" You'd laugh and say, "Stop hitting your foot with a hammer!" If you go to a licensed healthcare practitioner and say, "I have acid reflux. What do I do?" What you're really saying is, "Every time I load my body with the chemicals that the food industry is putting into our food supply, I get a burning sensation in my stomach." Well, the simple answer is: "Stop loading up your body with chemicals." Does this make sense?

A man came to me and said, "I have osteoporosis, what should I do?" My answer: "Let's figure out the cause of your osteoporosis. What's causing your body's inability to absorb sufficient calcium? Either (a) you're not getting enough calcium in your diet, or (b) something is blocking the absorption of calcium. It's really pretty simple isn't it?"

He said, "Yes."

I said, "Well, do you know the things that block calcium absorption?" He didn't know. I said, "Carbonated sodas. Do you drink a lot of them?"

His jaw almost hit the ground. He said, "I drink about ten a day."

"Well, if you're drinking ten a day, you're blocking your calcium absorption. It doesn't mean that's the reason for your osteoporosis, but it certainly could be."

I told my friend to visit a licensed healthcare practitioner and suggested that if he stopped drinking the carbonated sodas he would probably start absorbing calcium better. And so he did, and within a few months his condition corrected itself and he no longer had osteoporosis.

Somebody will say, "But not everyone who drinks carbonated sodas has osteoporosis." That's true, and not everyone who smokes cigarettes dies of lung cancer, but 90 percent of the people who die from lung cancer have smoked cigarettes. Get it?

> ...but more importantly, we're interested in learning what the cause of the symptoms is.

So, if you're experiencing some symptoms right now, our first goal is not to merely suppress those symptoms. Yes, we want them to go away, but more importantly, we're interested in learning what the cause of the symptoms is. We must also understand that since the symptoms did not develop overnight (they probably took years to develop), they may not vanish overnight, either. Like the example of the man hitting himself on the foot with the hammer, if we stop doing the thing that's causing the problem we still may have the current symptom for a while. Even if the man *stops* hitting his foot he may still have lingering pain. Why? Because he hit his foot with a hammer for so long he actually broke bones that need time to heal. Your medical condition may, similarly, need time to heal, before the symptoms subside entirely. So, understand that this approach requires patience.

If you find the cause of your problem while consulting with a licensed healthcare practitioner, together, you'll be able to address that cause. That's what this chapter is really all about.

Chapter 6 addresses the causes of ALL DISEASE. To review, those *causes* are: **(1) toxins in the body; (2) nutritional**

deficiencies; (3) electromagnetic chaos; and (4) emotional and mental stress. If you do all of the things in chapter 6 you'll address all four of these issues and thus be able to cure yourself of virtually any disease, and prevent future disease as well.

However, if you've done little to protect your health in twenty, thirty, forty, or fifty years, there's a good chance you have a serious situation that requires professional attention. This is why I state repeatedly that you must go to a licensed healthcare practitioner who does not only use drugs and surgery. Ideally you should see two or three different practitioners to get multiple opinions. When you go to your licensed healthcare practitioner and receive a personalized treatment for your situation, you can consider some of the following things. Remember, *I am not a doctor*; I have no medical training; I am not even a healthcare practitioner; I am not prescribing medical treatment; I am not treating any medical condition; I do not treat patients; and I am not making any attempt in this book to prescribe, diagnose, treat any illness, or treat any patient. I present this information simply for educational purposes only.

With that said, I'm going to present what I believe to be the best protocol to follow if you are currently sick. This is the procedure I would follow if I were to come down with an illness. Keep in mind that because I do the things in chapter 6, I never get sick.

Go back to chapter 6 and do all of the things recommended there.

I cannot emphasize this enough. The things that I mention in chapter 6, such as seeing a licensed healthcare practitioner, getting energetic rebalancing, doing all of the cleanses, etc. will, in my opinion, and in most cases, cure almost all diseases. Doing the things in chapter 6 can eliminate many, if not all, symptoms in a short period of time, because the recommendations address the root causes of all illness. Simply doing the energetic rebalancing and the various cleanses can cure the "incurable" by bringing the body back into balance. This has been documented by the million-plus reports from around the world confirming that these things effectively cure disease.

In addition to doing the things in chapter 6, there are some specific things you can do to help your body return to a state of "homeostasis" (balance), which will allow your body to heal itself faster. Remember, when given the right conditions, the body heals itself.

In addition to doing the things in chapter 6, I urge you to see a licensed healthcare practitioner. Getting individualized treatment from a licensed healthcare practitioner, which could include essential oils, herbs, homeopathic remedies, chiropractic care, vitamins, minerals, etc., can cure all disease. Getting energetic rebalancing and doing nothing else can virtually cure every disease. Doing a colon cleanse, liver/gallbladder cleanse, kidney cleanse, heavy metal cleanse, parasite cleanse, Candida cleanse, and a full-body cleanse can, in thirty to sixty days, cure any "incurable" disease. *Not* doing these things, in my opinion, makes trying to cure your disease much more difficult and next to impossible.

Yes, you could do some things to reduce your symptoms temporarily, or even eliminate them for a short time, but if you're not addressing the root cause they'll likely reoccur, or diseases will develop elsewhere in your body where there are genetic weaknesses. Therefore, if you want to cure yourself of the illness you have, you must get the toxins out of your body, and stop putting them in; you must start giving your body super nutrition; you must stop or at least neutralize the electromagnetic chaos that you're being exposed to; and you must eliminate any trapped emotional and/or mental stress that you're holding in your body unconsciously. Doing these things will change your body pH from acidic to alkaline where disease cannot exist.

Acid Reflux/Heartburn

Acid reflux is a condition in which food or liquid leaks backward from the stomach into the esophagus.

Main Cause	Natural Cures
Acid reflux can result from a number of issues including: Candida, parasites, nonprescription and prescription drugs, eating too much processed food, overeating, and mental and emotional stress.	• Take raw organic apple cider vinegar—2 to 4 tablespoons in 8 ounces of pure water before meals. • Take digestive enzymes—specifically with betaine hydrochloric acid. • Take probiotics—specifically acidophilus bifidus. • Do a Candida cleanse. • Do a parasite cleanse. • Do a colon cleanse. • Eat more organic raw fruits and vegetables. • Practice stress reduction. • Get alphabiotic alignment. • If symptoms worsen at night when you're reclining, try elevating the top your bed off the floor a couple of inches so that your upper body is lifted and the rest of your body slants down slightly.

Acne

A condition wherein sebaceous glands at the base of hair follicles in the pores of skin become inflamed or impacted with dead skin cells and a proliferation of acne causing bacteria, resulting in pimples.

Main Cause	Natural Cures
There are a number of factors that can result in acne. Some of these may include hormonal imbalances, bacteria in the digestive tract *and* on the skin, Candida, parasites, dehydration, allergies, a high-glycemic diet, and the use of oil-based makeup.	What causes one person's acne may be different for another, so if you're unable to control the condition on your own, see a naturopathic doctor who can evaluate you and determine the triggers specific to you. Two types of bacteria, *Propionibacterium acnes* and *Staphylococcus aureus*, can cause acne breakouts. Eliminating *P. acnes* and/or *S. aureus without* eliminating good bacteria is helpful in controlling acne. *Propionibacterium acnes* can be controlled in the digestive tract as well as topically.

Some suggestions:
- Drink 10 glasses of distilled water daily.
- Drink unsweetened aloe vera juice. (Kills *bad* bacteria.) Start with 2 ounces, build up to 6 ounces per day. Aloe vera juice has been shown to kill acne-causing bacteria in the digestive tract.
- Do a Candida cleanse.
- Do a colon cleanse.
- Do a liver/gallbladder cleanse.
- Do a parasite cleanse.
- Do a full-body fat cleanse.
- Exfoliate the skin regularly—skin brushing, microdermabrasion, and other forms of exfoliation can slough off the dead skin cells that may mix with sebum and contribute to clogged pores.
- Apply tea tree oil topically to affected areas.
- Internally, take 2 to 4 tablespoons of raw organic apple cider vinegar in 8 ounces of pure water before meals.
- Drink unsweetened, organic green tea (kills bad bacteria).
- Take probiotics.
- Take omega-3s.
- Eat organic plain yogurt (controls bad bacteria while maintaining good bacteria).
- Use an infrared sauna.
- Practice stress reduction.
- Eliminate sugar, white flour, milk products, and processed foods from the diet. These foods create acne-causing bacteria in the digestive tract.
- Coconut oil is an effective moisturizer for those suffering with acne breakouts. It is antibacterial and will not clog pores. Applying coconut oil will, over time, help *control* oily skin. While this seems counterintuitive, the reason is that the skin responds to the oil by minimizing its own production of oil.

ADD/ADHD

Attention deficit disorder (ADD) also known as attention deficit hyperactivity disorder (ADHD) is a persistent pattern of inattention and/or hyperactivity or impulsivity that is noticeably more frequent and severe than is typically observed in individuals at a comparable level of development.

Main Cause	Natural Cures
ADD and ADHD can result from a number of things including the presence of Candida in the body, ingesting food additives like monosodium glutamate, aspartame, and other artificial sweeteners, high fructose corn syrup, allergies, heavy metal toxicity, electromagnetic chaos, essential fatty acid deficiency, sensitivity to the chemicals in dairy and meat, nitrites, and blocked calcium absorption.	If you or your child has been diagnosed with ADD or ADHD, harsh medications may have been prescribed. See a naturopathic doctor for an evaluation and assistance in coming off harsh medications. While it can be difficult to change a child's diet dramatically, relief can come from dietary adjustments. Some suggestions: • Do a Candida cleanse. • Do a liver/gallbladder cleanse. • Take omega-3s. • Eliminate dairy. • Eliminate nitrites. • Eliminate high fructose corn syrup. • Eliminate artificial sweeteners. • Eliminate fast food. • Get alphabiotic alignment (alleviates stress). • Get cranial sacral therapy. • Practice stress reduction.

Allergies

An allergy is an immune response to something that either enters the body, or comes in contact with the body and causes hypersensitivity. The substance is usually harmless, however in sensitive individuals, the body responds to the substance as if it were a pathogen and tries to destroy it.

Main Cause	Natural Cures
Allergies are caused by a variety of things that are specific to individuals. Triggers may include a weakened immune system, Candida, clogged liver, weak adrenal glands, and lack of exposure to irritants in early childhood.	Though allergic reactions are unique to the individual, in using natural cures the first goal should be to assist the body in ways that will reduce its tendency to produce antibodies that result in allergic reactions. See a licensed naturopathic doctor who can assist you in strengthening your adrenal, digestive, and immune systems.

Some suggestions:

- Drink 10, 8-ounce glasses of distilled water daily.
- Do a liver/gallbladder cleanse.
- Do a Candida cleanse.
- Do a colon cleanse.
- Consult with a certified NAET practitioner. (NAET is an allergy elimination technique.)
- Practice stress reduction.
- Take bee pollen (do *not* take if you're allergic to bees or pollen).
- Take bioflavonoids.
- Take flaxseed oil.
- Take probiotics.
- Take the herbs dong quai and gingko biloba.
- Dietary adjustments: eliminate alcohol, caffeine, artificial food colorings, processed sugar and wheat.
- Eat: leafy greens, yellow vegetables, onions, garlic, ginger, cayenne, and kimchi.

Anxiety/Stress

Stress can be the result of a situation that is frustrating, or that provokes anger, or creates nervousness. Anxiety is the feeling of intense worry, unease, or fear.

Main Cause	Natural Cures
The cause of anxiety and/or stress is unique to each individual. However, there are physiological conditions that can contribute to stress and anxiety. For example, many people report feeling relief from stress and anxiety after doing a fast or a cleanse, which would suggest that diet and the state of the body can contribute to, or exacerbate stress and anxiety.	• See one or more licensed healthcare practitioners. Consider a chiropractor, herbalist, acupuncturist, hypnotist, Thought Field Therapy specialist (Callahan technique), or Emotional Freedom Technique specialist. • Practice stress reduction. • Get alphabiotic alignment. • Get massages. • Exercise. • Meditate. • Do rebounding.

	• Walk for an hour each day.
	• Drive less.
	• Don't talk on a cell phone and drive.
	• Get adequate sunlight.
	• Get adequate rest.
	• Reduce usage of cell phones, computers, tablets etc.
	• Reduce or eliminate caffeine. Excess caffeine can cause an anxiety attack.
	• Do an organic juice fast.
	• Do a heavy metal cleanse.
	• Do a colon cleanse.
	• Do a liver/gallbladder cleanse.

Arthritis

Arthritis is degeneration or inflammation and/or stiffness of the joints.

Main Cause	Natural Cures
Arthritis can result from loss of collagen, Candida, heavy metal toxicity, parasites, and viruses.	See a naturopathic doctor who can determine the specific type of arthritis you have (there are over a hundred types), and then create a plan to address it. In some cases herbs may be beneficial. If your naturopath doesn't prescribe herbs, you may want to visit an herbalist. Homeopathy may benefit the condition as well. A "homeopathic" doctor is different from a naturopathic doctor, although some naturopaths practice homeopathy. Anti-inflammatory drugs which may have provided pain relief can actually reduce the body's ability to repair cartilage and make the condition worse, so you will need to stop taking over-the-counter pain killers if you've been using them. Some suggestions: • Drink 8 to 10 glasses of pure water daily. • Eliminate foods in the "nightshade" family: tomatoes, potatoes, peppers, eggplant and tobacco. These contain alkaloids that can increase inflammation.

	• Eliminate: sugar, processed foods, caffeine. • Eat: kale, celery, mustard greens, almonds, figs, limes, olive oil, unflavored gelatin. • Supplements: cetyl myristoleate (CMO), dimethyl sulfoxide (DMSO), methyl-sulfonylmethane (MSM), glucosamine, copper, evening primrose oil, royal jelly, omega-5e, SierraSil, flaxseed oil. • Herbs: black cohosh, burdock, larrea, devil's claw. • Homeopathy: Bryonia, Ruta graveolens. • Do a parasite cleanse. • Take crocodile protein peptide. • Drink organic bone broth (provides collagen). • Use castor oil packs (cotton flannel soaked in castor oil, placed on the body with a heating pad or hot water bottle on top). • Remove all metal from the mouth.

Asthma

A disorder wherein the airways of the lungs swell and narrow, leading to wheezing, shortness of breath, chest tightness, and coughing.

Main Cause	Natural Cures
A number of circumstances can lead to asthma, including trapped mental and emotional stress, allergies, hormonal imbalance, Candida, lack of early exposure to bacteria preventing immune system stimulation, environmental irritants, poor diet, reaction to lactose, having been fed a breast milk substitute in infancy that was an allergen, use of antibiotics in early childhood, insufficient stomach acid production.	See a naturopathic doctor who can develop a comprehensive approach to the condition. Rather than plying you with drugs that only treat the symptoms, a good N.D. will work on a variety of aspects of the condition. These may include reducing allergic exposure, reducing the sensitivity and spasticity of the airways of the lungs, addressing nutritional deficiencies and imbalances, and addressing the inflammatory pathways of the body. Some suggestions: • Do a colon cleanse. • Do a Candida cleanse. • Do a liver cleanse. • Do a heavy metal cleanse.

	• Remove metal from the mouth. • Eliminate wheat. • Take probiotics. • Supplements: hyrdrochloric acid (helps replace stomach acid often lacking in asthma sufferers), magnesium, omega-3s, vitamin C, vitamin B6. • Avoid cow's milk and high lactose products. • Practice stress reduction. • Do oxygen therapy.

Autism

A systemic body disorder affecting the brain with developmental disabilities that appear within the first three years of life. Social and communication skills are impaired.

Main Cause	Natural Cures
Autism is a complicated disorder, which may result from environmental toxins, genetics (the toxins trigger a genetic response in those susceptible), viral infections, heavy metal toxicity, mercury, Candida, and adverse reaction to prescription and nonprescription drugs.	Find a naturopathic doctor who specializes in treating autism. An N.D. will likely recommend detoxification of heavy metals, viruses and bacteria, and once the detox has been achieved, further treatment may include neurological healing. Recommendations: • Heavy metal cleanse, Candida cleanse, colon cleanse. • Drink pure, un-fluoridated water. • Test for food allergens and eliminate those allergens from your diet. • Eliminate processed foods. • Eliminate GMOs. • Take probiotics. • Take digestive enzymes. Vaccines are the controversial culprits in autism. According to medical science the theory that vaccines cause the disorder has been debunked. However, there are people who continue to believe that vaccines do contribute to autism in children who are genetically predisposed to mercury sensitivity.

Back Pain

Back pain usually originates from the muscles, nerves, bones, joints or other structures in the spine.

Main Cause	Natural Cures
Mental and emotional stress, trauma, dehydration, viral infections, improper posture, and movements that lead to misalignment can all contribute to back pain.	• See a chiropractor and/or an acupuncturist; both can be especially helpful with back pain. • Drink 8 glasses of pure water daily. • Get alphabiotic alignment. • Get rolfing. • Get cranial sacral therapy. • Get deep-tissue massage. • Use a magnetic mattress pad. • Practice stress reduction.

Bad Breath

Chronic unpleasant odor of the breath that is not due to something one has eaten.

Main Cause	Natural Cures
Lack of digestive enzymes, toxic overload, Candida, parasites, heavy metal toxicity, prescription and nonprescription drugs, constipation, and a sluggish liver are among the many contributing factors to bad breath.	A change in diet to include more raw fruits and vegetables and eliminating processed foods will help with this condition. People who eat high protein diets with a lot of meat and few live foods will tend to have bad breath. Some suggestions: • Drink at least 8 glasses of pure water daily. • Do a colon cleanse. • Take digestive enzymes. • Do a liver/gallbladder cleanse. • Do a Candida cleanse. • Drink aloe vera juice. • Take organic raw apple cider vinegar in pure water (2 to 4 tablespoons in 8 ounces) twice daily. • Take probiotics. • Use an infrared sauna. • Drink green juice containing parsley or cilantro, which acts as a deodorizer.

Bladder Infection
A bacterial infection in the urinary tract, also called cystitis.

Main Cause	Natural Cures
When germs or bacteria enter through the urethra the result may be a bladder or urinary tract infection.	If you're experiencing recurring symptoms see a naturopathic doctor. Without proper treatment, bladder infections can lead to more serious conditions. Some suggestions: • Alkalize urine by drinking 1/2 teaspoon of baking soda in 8 ounces of pure water. • Take raw organic apple cider vinegar (2 tablespoons) mixed with 1 tablespoon of raw honey in 8 ounces two to three times daily before meals. • Drink organic *unsweetened* pure cranberry juice (up to a quart a day)—best if made fresh with a juicer at home. Cranberry juice is very strong; dilute with pure water as necessary, or juice with another organic fruit like apples: one part apple to two parts cranberries. • Homeopathic remedies can be helpful. See a homeopathic doctor for treatment. Some homeopathic remedies to consider include Belladonna, Berberis Vulgaris, Cantharis, and sarsaparilla. • Take larrea. • Take bee propolis.

Bloating/Gas
Feeling that the abdomen is enlarged, sometimes includes actual intermittent distention of the abdomen generally caused by intestinal gas.

Main Cause	Natural Cures
There are many things that can cause gas, including intestinal bacteria, Candida, parasites, nonprescription and prescription drugs, processed foods, sugars (lactose, sorbitol, fructose in particular), artificial sweeteners	Chronic gas can signal a more serious issue with your digestive tract, so visit a naturopathic doctor if your bloating/gas persists after eliminating what you believe to be the source. Some suggestions: • Take digestive enzymes with betaine hydrochloric acid.

<table>
<tr><td>(especially mannitol and xylitol), polysaccharides (wheat in particular), fruits and vegetable that are high in sugar and/or polysaccharides.</td><td>

• Take raw organic apple cider, 2 to 4 tablespoons in 8 ounces of pure water before meals.

• Eliminate wheat.

• Eliminate sugars and artificial sweeteners that cause a reaction.

• Drink aloe vera juice, 4 ounces before breakfast.

• Drink ginger tea: peel and chop a large piece of ginger, boil in a pot of,16 to 20 ounces of water, cool and drink the "ginger tea."

• Take liquid sage in pure water.

• Take probiotics.

• Do a Candida cleanse.

• Do a parasite cleanse.

• Do a colon cleanse.
</td></tr>
</table>

Blood Clots

Blood clots are abnormally formed semi-solid masses of coagulated blood. They can be life threatening.

Main Cause	Natural Cures
Blood clots can result from nonprescription and prescription drug use, mental and emotional stress, trans fats (hydrogenated oils), homogenized dairy products, vitamin E deficiency, obesity, and being immobile for long periods of time, for example on long flights or drives.	See a naturopathic doctor if you've been diagnosed with a blood clot, if you suspect that you have one, or know that you're prone to them. Some suggestions: • Take raw apple cider vinegar, 2 to 4 ounces in 8 ounces of pure water, add a dash of cayenne pepper. • Add ginger to your diet. • Walk daily. • Take natural vitamin E. • Take nattokinase. • Take oral chelation. (Both nattokinase and oral chelation improve circulation.)

Cancer	
An uncontrolled growth of abnormal cells in the body.	
Main Cause	**Natural Cures**
Cancer results from toxins in the body, nutritional deficiencies, electromagnetic chaos, mental and emotional stress.	See a licensed healthcare practitioner. Start with a naturopathic doctor. An N.D. may recommend other healthcare practitioners to assist with your treatment. Some suggestions: • Do all of the things recommended in chapter 6. It's very important that you eliminate toxins, improve your body's ability to absorb nutrients, eliminate electromagnetic chaos and eliminate stress. • Drink fresh, unpasteurized, organic juices made with low-sugar vegetables and low-sugar fruits. • Eat more raw fruits (low-glycemic) and vegetables. (Improves your nutritional intake.) • Eliminate sugars, including natural sugars from the diet. Fructose promotes the growth of cancer cells. • Eliminate processed vegetable oils. (Soy, corn, canola, and margarine are chemically altered and toxic to the body.) • Take omega-3s. • Take vitamin D. • Take linseed oil. • Take food grade hydrogen peroxide (35%). • Take oxygen therapy. • See a specialist in Chinese medicine. • Practice stress reduction. Laugh, get massages, meditate, and walk in nature. • Get plenty of sleep.

Cardiac Arrhythmia
Irregular heartbeat.

Main Cause	Natural Cures
A weakened or damaged heart, excessive caffeine, smoking, alcohol abuse, drug abuse, and mental stress can all cause cardiac arrhythmia.	See a licensed healthcare practitioner, beginning with a naturopathic doctor. This can be a serious condition and not one that's appropriate for self-treatment. Some recommendations: • Get acupuncture. • Take fish oil. • Take magnesium—tends to stabilize the heart. • Take potassium. • Take vitamin C. • Take the herb hawthorn berry. • Avoid caffeine. • Take nattokinase. (Improves circulation, strengthens the heart.) • Reduce stress.

Chemical Sensitivity
Multiple chemical sensitivity (MCS) is a response to chemical, biological or physical agents, manifesting in a number of symptoms including headache, fatigue, nausea, diarrhea, muscle pain, sneezing, itching, sore throat, rashes, gas, bloating, confusion, concentration and memory problems and mood swings. These responses can be due to chemical spills, or to things as minor as new carpet, bedding, ventilation systems, cleaning products, perfumes, automobile exhaust or anything with some sort of chemical residue.

Main Cause	Natural Cures
Toxic chemicals are generally the cause, although some believe that there's an immune response similar to allergies that causes people with the condition to be highly sensitive to low levels of chemicals deemed safe and that do not cause discomfort in others.	• Detox—to rid your body of any ingested toxins. • Do all of the cleanses recommended in chapter 6. • Stop using any chemical cleaners. • Avoid plastics in food preparation. • Use air purifiers with HEPA filters. • Use a vacuum with a HEPA filter.

Chronic Fatigue Syndrome (CFS)

Extreme fatigue that doesn't improve with rest, often accompanies by achiness and swollen lymph nodes.

Main Cause	Natural Cures
CFS may be caused by Candida, viruses—in particular the Epstein-Barr virus, parasites, heavy metal toxicity, hypoactive thyroid, and allergies.	• Do all of the things in chapter 6. • Test body pH and if too acid, alkalize the body. • Practice yoga and/or meditation. • See a homeopathic doctor. Homeopathic remedies may include muriatic acid, Gelsemium, Kali Phosphoricum, picric acid, and Stannum. • Eliminate wheat. • Eliminate caffeine. • Eliminate alcohol. • Eat raw foods. • Eat/use extra virgin coconut oil—use in cooking and mix into fruit/vegetable smoothies.

Crohn's Disease

Crohn's is a form of inflammatory bowel disease that involves the intestines, but may affect any part of the gastrointestinal tract and range anywhere from the mouth to the anus.

Main Cause	Natural Cures
What causes Crohn's is unclear, but diet and stress aggravate the situation. In people with Crohn's the immune system responds to normal bacteria like harmful invaders and produces chronic inflammation in the intestines.	Some suggestions: • See a naturopathic doctor who can evaluate you and create a treatment plan specifically designed for you. • Acupuncture is helpful for some Crohn's sufferers. • Take probiotics, specifically acidophilus and bifidus organisms, which help restore healthy bacteria to the intestines. • Take fish oil. • Consider biofeedback treatment, which has been shown to improve the condition in some. • Drink aloe vera juice.

	• Eliminate gluten.
	• Eliminate lactose.
	• Avoid fried foods.
	• Reduce caffeine consumption.
	• Reduce alcohol consumption.

Circulation Problems

Restricted blood flow in the body that can lead to more serious conditions.

Main Cause	Natural Cures
Blockages in the arteries due to chlorine in drinking and/ or bathing water, homogenized dairy products, trans fats, Candida, heavy metals, allergies and viruses can all contribute to circulation problems.	See a naturopathic doctor who can evaluate the causes for your particular circulation issues. Some suggestions: • Drink at least 8 glasses of pure water daily. Filter your drinking water and bathing water. • Avoid chlorinated pools. • Avoid dairy that is pasteurized and homogenized. • Take oral chelation. • For severe cases take intravenous chelation. • Take food grade hydrogen peroxide therapy (35%). • Take natural vitamin E. • Take omega-3s. • Get massages. • Walk for an hour daily.

Cold Sores

Often called "fever blisters," they are small sores that appear on the lips or outer edges of the mouth. Also known as herpes simplex virus type 1 (HSV-1).

Main Cause	Natural Cures
Viral infection is the cause of cold sores. If you've had the chicken pox, you have been exposed to HSV-1. (Not the same virus that causes genital herpes.)	See a licensed healthcare provider. A naturopathic doctor, a homeopathic doctor and an herbalist all may be helpful in controlling and even eradicating the condition. (Despite medical science's claim that there is no cure.) Some suggestions: • Do all of the things recommended in chapter 6, particularly the cleanses.

- Strengthen the immune system; a weakened immune system is what allows the virus to attack.
- Some suggestions for immune support:
- Take echinacea, vitamin C and zinc.
- Take reishi mushroom.
- Take larrea.
- Take red marine algae.
- Take lysine.
- Take food grade hydrogen peroxide (35%).
- Use dimethyl sulfoxide (DMSO) topically to heal lesions.
- Consider the following anti-viral herbs: thyme, lapacho, astragalus, licorice, galangal, cat's claw, ligustrum, pansy, cayenne and myrrh. These are suggestions, but rather than self-prescribing, see a professional herbalist who can determine which of these is best for your particular situation.
- Homeopathic remedies to consider include Natrum muriaticum, Rhus toxicodendron and Sepia. Again, rather than self-medicate, get an evaluation from a trained herbalist.

With all of these suggestions, you must first do the things in chapter 6. You need to bring your body into balance and remove toxins from your system before any treatment will eradicate the virus.

Colds

Common viral infection affecting the upper respiratory system, wherein the mucus membranes of the throat and nose become inflamed.

Main Cause	Natural Cures
Colds are the result of a viral infection, usually the "rhinovirus," which infiltrates the cells that line the nasal passages and then proliferates.	If you do the things in chapter 6 you should not come down with colds. It's possible to go for years without contracting viruses if the immune system is strong and the body's pH is alkaline. Some suggestions: • Bed rest.

	• Make a nasal spray or flush with pure warm water, sea salt and baking soda. Mix 1 teaspoon of sea salt, 1 teaspoon of baking soda, and 1 cup of warm water in a bowl. You can inhale it drawing the water into your nose, which is not comfortable, but will help clear congestion. OR, you can use a bulb syringe and spray it into your nose. • Take Oscillococcinum—a homeopathic remedy that's easy to find in drugs stores. • Take green papaya extract. • Take digestive enzymes. • Take probiotics. • Take crocodile protein peptide. • Use an infrared sauna. • Get sunlight. • Drink ginger tea made with raw ginger boiled in water.

Colitis

Colitis is a swelling of the large intestine.

Main Cause	Natural Cures
People of Ashkenazi heritage are more prone to colitis leading to the conclusion that genetics may play quite a large role in the condition. However, lifestyle choices are also a factor. Poor diet—sugars, processed foods, wheat, white flour, and too much linoleic acid which is found in red meat, margarine, processed foods and vegetable oils including soybean oil, corn oil, and safflower oil, can lead to colitis.	See a naturopathic doctor who can put together a program specifically for you. Some suggestions: • Drink aloe vera juice. The amount will vary from person to person. Aloe vera juice has an anti-inflammatory effect on the intestine. • Take probiotics. • Take omega-3s. • Take boswellia extract. • Do a Candida cleanse. • Eliminate sugar. • Eliminate wheat. • Eliminate flour (white and whole wheat). • Take bromelain. • Practice stress reduction.

Constipation

A condition where there is difficulty emptying the bowels and one may experience bowel movements less than three times per week and with hardened stools.

Main Cause	Natural Cures
A number of lifestyle choices will result in conditions that cause constipation. Eating food without living enzymes, white flour, white sugar and refined foods that cause poor gut flora, Candida, taking nonprescription and prescription drugs, not eating enough fibrous foods, mental and emotional stress, and not drinking enough water (dehydration) all contribute to constipation.	Short-term constipation can be addressed on one's own, but long-term or chronic constipation is serious and requires the help of a licensed healthcare practitioner such as a naturopathic doctor. Doing the recommendations in chapter 6 will alleviate constipation. Some suggestions: • Drink 10 glasses of distilled water daily. • Eat 5 organic apples a day. • Eat prunes. • Eat ginger—raw in smoothies and/or cooked in vegetable stir-fry dishes. • Get colonics. • Drink aloe vera juice. • Drink 2 to 4 tablespoons of raw organic apple cider vinegar in 8 ounces of pure water before meals. • Take probiotics. • Take digestive enzymes. • Do a colon cleanse. • Do a Candida cleanse.

Cough

Coughing is a natural reflex that protects the lungs, however a prolonged or persistent cough can indicate infection or disease.

Main Cause	Natural Cures
Candida, bacterial or viral infections, and allergies may cause coughs.	• Gargle with warm water (pure or distilled) and sea salt. • Gargle with colloidal minerals. • Drink hot tea with organic lemon and raw honey. • Make a mixture of melted coconut oil, raw honey (1 tablespoon of each) and 1/2 an organic lemon and sip slowly letting it coat the throat.

Dandruff

Dandruff is a scalp condition in which skin flakes off. It can be due to dry scalp or it can be due to eczema, psoriasis, seborrheic dermatitis, or fungal infection.

Main Cause	Natural Cures
Dandruff can result from a number of things including Candida, toxic overload, allergies, dehydration and parasites.	• Wash the scalp with baking soda (mix one part baking soda with two parts water and pour over the scalp, follow with a rinse made of equal parts of raw apple cider vinegar and water and then rinse with water thoroughly. • You can also mix equal parts raw apple cider vinegar and pure water, add to a spray bottle, spray on the scalp and allow it to sit for 20 minutes and then wash out. • Massage scalp with extra virgin coconut oil, leave in either for 15 minutes or overnight and wash out the next day. • Do all of the cleanses recommended in chapter 6. • Take probiotics. • Take omega-3s. • Drink 10 glasses of distilled water daily.

Depression

Feelings of severe despondency accompanied by feelings of hopelessness and inadequacy that persists over a period of time.

Main Cause	Natural Cures
The causes of depression are unique to each individual. Candida can contribute to depression in some people. Poor diet, poor sleep habits, chronic dehydration, and hormonal imbalance can also contribute to depression.	• See a licensed healthcare practitioner for a treatment plan specifically designed for you. A naturopathic doctor can advise on natural remedies as well as make recommendations for other kinds of therapies. • See an acupuncturist. • Suggested supplements: St. John's wort, S-Adenosylmethionine (SAM-E), omega-3s. Some suggestions: • Get adequate sleep. • Walk for an hour daily.

	• Spend more time in the sun, 20 minutes per day when possible.
	• Do rebounding.
	• Eliminate all prescription and nonprescription drugs.
	• Eliminate aspartame.
	• Drink 8 to10 glasses of pure water daily.
	• Do a Candida cleanse.
	• Do all of the cleanses recommended in chapter 6.
	• Do a week-long juice fast using fresh, organic, non-pasteurized low-sugar vegetables and fruits.
	• Practice stress reduction.
	• Do Thought Field Therapy (TFT) or the Emotional Freedom Technique (EFT).

Diabetes

A metabolic disease in which the body's inability to produce insulin results in high levels of sugar (or glucose) in the blood.

Main Cause	Natural Cures
Genetics *and* behavioral factors play a part diabetes, type 1 and type 2. Type 1, early onset, seems to be inherited, while type 2 appears to result primarily from lifestyle choices. Prescription drugs, Candida, artificial sweeteners, too much white sugar and white flour, trans fats, obesity, and being sedentary contribute to type 2 diabetes, but because the disease may run in families some believe there may be a genetic link there as well. Though, generally this can be attributed to the dietary and exercise	See a naturopathic doctor who can develop a plan for you. Type 1 and type 2 diabetes can be treated successfully. Some suggestions: • Lose weight if you're overweight. • Eliminate aspartame. It's toxic and makes weight loss more difficult. • Eliminate all prescription and nonprescription drugs. • Eliminate all processed foods. • Eliminate sugar and white flour. • Reduce consumption of grains. • Consume raw vegetables and low-glycemic fruits. • Eat probiotic foods: kimchi, sauerkraut, organic plain yogurt.

habits in families being similar. Doing the things in chapter 6 will help both forms of diabetes.	• Consider adding these to the diet: cinnamon, ginger, aloe vera, and bilberry extract. • Take omega-3s. • Take vitamin C. • Take vitamin D—cod liver oil is a good source. • Walk for an hour daily. • Do a Candida cleanse.

Diarrhea

A condition involving the frequent passing of loose or watery stools.

Main Cause	Natural Cures
Parasites, Candida, prescription and nonprescription drugs, flu virus, and bacteria are all causes of diarrhea.	• Drink 8 to 10 glasses of distilled water daily. • Take digestive enzymes. • Take fenugreek seeds. • Take probiotics. • Eat probiotics, in particular, organic plain yogurt with active cultures. • Do a Candida cleanse. • Do a parasite cleanse. • Do a colon cleanse. • Do a liver/gallbladder cleanse.

Eczema

Eczema is a skin condition wherein patches of skin become rough and inflamed with blisters that cause itching and bleeding.

Main Cause	Natural Cures
Eczema is believed to be a genetically inherited condition. Allergies, hormonal imbalance, and stress can trigger flare-ups.	• Do all of the things in chapter 6. • See a naturopathic doctor. • Homeopathy, hypnosis and acupuncture should also be explored as all have been helpful among eczema sufferers. Some suggestions: • Eliminate wheat and all gluten. • Consider eliminating milk, eggs, nuts and soy, which can be triggers. • Take gamma-linolenic acid (GMA).

- Take evening primrose oil.
- Take fish oil.
- Take vitamin A.
- Take vitamin B complex.
- Take vitamin E.
- Take zinc.
- Take the Bach flower essence Rescue Remedy (drops). Rescue Remedy also comes in a topical ointment that may be applied to the affected areas.
- Use aloe vera gel topically.
- Use coconut oil topically as a lotion.
- Practice stress reduction.

Edema

Edema is fluid retention that leads to bloating or swelling in the body's tissues.

Main Cause	Natural Cures
There are a number of causes for edema, including general lack of physical activity, standing or sitting for too long, surgery, burns, menstruation, menopause, prescription and nonprescription drugs, and poor diet. A number of illnesses and conditions can cause edema as well, including head injury, heart failure, diabetes, allergies, arthritis, liver disease, kidney disease, thyroid disease and chronic lung disease.	• Do all of the things in chapter 6. • See a naturopathic doctor. Some recommendations: • Take dandelion leaf (a natural diuretic). • Take vitamin B complex. • Take vitamin C. • Take vitamin D. • Take pantothenic acid. • Take potassium. • Reduce salt intake.

Fibromyalgia

A syndrome in which there is long-term body-wide pain and tenderness in the joints, muscles, tendons and other soft tissues.

Main Cause	Natural Cures
Causes vary from person to person. Stress and toxic overload can contribute to	• See a naturopathic doctor who can determine the cause of your fibromyalgia and create a treatment plan specifically for you.

| the condition. Some people develop fibromyalgia after an accident or trauma. | • Do all of the cleanses in chapter 6.
• Eliminate wheat, dairy, sugar and processed foods.
• Take oral chelation.
• Take crocodile protein peptide.
• Use a magnetic mattress pad. |

Gallbladder Problems

Most gallbladder issues are due to inflammation of the organ resulting when gallstones obstruct the ducts leading to the small intestines.

Main Cause	Natural Cures
Prescription and nonprescription drugs, excessive intake of trans fats, Candida, genetic weaknesses exacerbated by chemicals in food (primarily meat and dairy), food allergies, hypothyroidism, and lack of exercise all contribute to gallbladder issues.	See a naturopathic doctor for a treatment plan. Some suggestions: • Do a liver/gallbladder cleanse. • Do a heavy metal cleanse. • Do a Candida cleanse. • Do a colon cleanse. • Do a parasite cleanse. • Do a heavy metal cleanse. • Take digestive enzymes.

Gout

A type of arthritis that occurs when uric acid builds up in the blood and leads to inflammation of the joints, or often one joint in particular.

Main Cause	Natural Cures
Eating too many foods rich in "purines." Organ meats are particularly high in purines. Other causes include consuming high fructose corn syrup, excess protein in the blood, poor circulation, being overweight, and excessive alcohol consumption. Some people are genetically predisposed to gout. Some prescription and nonprescription drugs can cause gout such as diuretics, aspirin, cyclosporine, and levodopa.	• Lose weight if you're overweight. • Drink 8 to 10 glasses of pure water daily. (Will assist the body in flushing out uric acid.) • Eliminate alcohol. • Eliminate organ meats and high fructose corn syrup. • Exercise regularly. • Eat organic strawberries. Strawberries help the body get rid of excess uric acid. • Both oral and intravenous chelation therapy can help with gout.

Heart Disease

Any type of disorder that affects the heart. It is distinct from cardiovascular disease, which affects disorders of the blood vessels *and* the heart. Heart disease refers only to the heart. More specifically, these diseases include angina (heart muscle doesn't get enough oxygen), arrhythmia (irregular heartbeat), congenital (birth defects of the heart), coronary artery disease (diseased coronary arteries), dilated cardiomyopathy (heart chambers dilated due to weak heart muscle), myocardial infarction (heart attack or interrupted blood flow), heart failure (heart doesn't pump blood around the body efficiently), hypertrophic cardiomyopathy (wall of left ventricle too thick, making it harder for blood to leave the heart), mitral regurgitation (when mitral valve doesn't close tightly enough and blood flows back into the heart), mitral valve prolapse (when valve between left atrium and left ventricle does not fully close; it bulges upwards back into the atrium), pulmonary stenosis (when pulmonary valve is too tight making it difficult for the heart to pump blood from the right ventricle to the pulmonary artery).

Main Cause	Natural Cures
Smoking, being overweight, excess sugar consumption (damages the arteries), Candida, bacterial infections, viral infections, parasites, heavy metal toxicity, trans fats, homogenized dairy products, chlorinated drinking and bathing water, nonprescription and prescription drugs, lack of exercise, magnesium deficiency, and mental and emotional stress can all contribute to heart disease.	See a naturopathic doctor to devise a plan specifically for you. Some suggestions: • Weight loss if needed. Being overweight strains the heart. • Eat a primarily plant-based diet. If your arteries have plaque, eliminate the foods that contributed to that. • Eliminate processed meats. • Exercise regularly to get your heart rate up. 30 minutes per day—walk, rebound, dance— *move.* • Eliminate processed foods and sugar. In recent years, a connection between sugar's inflammatory effect and artery damage has been discovered. • Take probiotics. Heart disease has been linked to unhealthy gut flora. You can also eat probiotic foods such as kimchi, sauerkraut, and plain organic yogurt. • Take omega-3s. • Take natural vitamin E. • Take magnesium.

| | • Take oral chelation and in extreme cases intravenous chelation, which will improve circulation. |

Hepatitis C
A viral disease that leads to inflammation of the liver.

Main Cause	Natural Cures
Hepatitis C is a viral infection one can contract via sharing needles with someone who has the virus. It is generally contracted when one is exposed to contaminated blood. Years ago, people receiving blood transfusions were at risk, however, blood used for transfusion is now screened for hepatitis C to prevent spread of the condition.	• If you have hepatitis C see an herbalist and/or an expert in Chinese medicine. • Herbal treatments may include milk thistle, schizandra, bupleurum, scutellaria, isatis, licorice root, astragalus, and white peony.

Herpes
A viral infection affecting the skin. We discussed cold sores (type 1) above. Type 2 is genital herpes.

Main Cause	Natural Cures
Genital herpes results from contact with someone who has the virus.	See a healthcare practitioner who can evaluate you and develop a treatment plan specifically for you. Consider a naturopathic doctor, an herbalist, and/or homeopathic doctor. Some suggestions: • Detox. Do a colon cleanse, a Candida cleanse, a liver and gallbladder cleanse. This will strengthen your immune system. A weakened immune system allows the virus to flare up. • Remedy nutritional deficiencies. Consider a fresh, organic juice fast. • Eat raw, organic fruits and vegetables. • Address energetic frequency imbalances. Homeopathy deals with frequencies.

	• Consider an energetic balancing program. With the AIM program (www.AIMprogram.com) you can have your energetic frequencies balanced twenty-four hours a day.
	• Take lysine. Lysine is an amino acid that helps suppress the virus.
	• Take red marine algae. This product appears to eliminate the herpes virus.
	• Use dimethyl sulfoxide (DMSO). Applied topically, it kills the virus.
	• Take food grade hydrogen peroxide therapy (35%).
	• Drink liquid oxygen. The virus cannot live in an oxygen rich environment.
	• Take larrea. This plant is anti-viral and can kill the herpes virus in 30 days.
	• Herbal remedies include thyme, lapacho, astragalus, licorice, galangal, cat's claw, ligustrum, pansy, cayenne, and myrrh.
	• Homeopathic remedies include Natrum muriaticum, Rhus toxicodendron, and Sepia.

High Blood Pressure
When blood pressure is 140/90 or higher most of the time.

Main Cause	Natural Cures
Mental and emotional stress, nutritional deficiencies, a diet high in sodium, a diet high in fructose, Candida, being overweight, and smoking all contribute to high blood pressure.	• Do a Candida cleanse.
	• Eliminate processed sugar, white flower, white rice, and white potatoes. These foods elevate insulin levels and also keep blood pressure elevated.
	• Eliminate caffeine. Caffeine exacerbates hypertension.
	• Take omega-3s—fish oil, flaxseed.
	• Take natural vitamin E.
	• Take calcium and magnesium. (Both have been shown to lower blood pressure.)
	• Eat organic extra virgin coconut oil.

	• Reduce omega-6s (corn oil, soy oil, canola oil.)
	• Consume probiotic fermented foods such as kimchi, sauerkraut, natto, miso, organic, plain yogurt. Bad bacteria in the gut is linked to heart disease.
	• Get more vitamin D via sun exposure. (Helps regulate blood pressure.)
	• Exercise—walk daily.
	• Practice stress reduction.

High Cholesterol
The presence of high levels of fats in the blood.

Main Cause	Natural Cures
For some, genetics play a part in high cholesterol. For others, it's lifestyle choices—eating too many foods that are high in saturated fats and trans fats, smoking, stress, being overweight and being sedentary.	• Doing the things in chapter 6 can help those with a genetic predisposition to high cholesterol as well as those afflicted as a result of behavioral choices.
	• See a naturopathic doctor who can pre-scribe a treatment plan specifically for you.
	Some suggestions:
	• Eliminate foods high in saturated fat such as red meat, processed meat, most cheese, and lard.
	• Eliminate pastry, cakes, biscuits, cream, and anything with trans fats.
	• Eat more raw foods—organic fruits and vegetables.
	• Eat more whole grains, particularly oats, which reduce cholesterol.
	• Eat good quality fats with omega-3s—fish oil, walnuts, hemp seeds, and chia seeds.
	• Eat garlic.
	• Replace corn oil and soy oil with olive oil. Coconut oil is also a good oil for cook-ing and contrary to what was previously believed, coconut oil does not raise choles-terol.
	• Take garlic supplements.
	• Take red yeast rice.

	• Drink mangosteen juice.
	• Lose weight if overweight.
	• Exercise regularly.
	• Avoid excessive alcohol. Red wine in moderation, however, is helpful in reducing cholesterol.
	• Stop smoking.
	• Practice stress reduction.

Inflammation/Pain (chronic)

Inflammation is the body's attempt to remove harmful stimuli, including damaged cells, and/or pathogens and begin the healing process.

Main Cause	Natural Cures
Inflammation is the body's response to infection or injury. *Chronic* inflammation is an over-response resulting from a variety of issues that may include dehydration and blockage of electromagnetic impulses between cells.	• See a licensed healthcare practitioner who can treat your pain without pharmaceutical drugs. Pharmaceutical pain medications are highly addictive and harmful. • Depending on the source of your inflammation, acupuncture can be especially helpful. • Chiropractic adjustments are also recommended. Some suggestions: • Drink 10 glasses of pure water a day. • Use a magnetic mattress pad. • Get alphabiotic adjustments. • Do a Candida cleanse. • Do a heavy metal cleanse. • Take oral chelation. • Do ozone therapy.

Insomnia

Persistent difficulty falling asleep, or staying asleep through the night.

Main Cause	Natural Cures
Many different things result in insomnia and each person's cause may be different from the next. Among the many triggers are anxiety/stress, excess caffeine, alcohol	• Practice stress reduction, including relaxation exercises, and deep breathing. • Meditate. • Get massages.

| consumed too close to bedtime, hormonal imbalance, lack of exercise, pain, prescription and nonprescription drugs, electronics in the bedroom, and medical conditions. | • Exercise regularly, preferably daily. Walk for one hour a day.
• Eliminate prescription and nonprescription medication.
• Do a Candida cleanse.
• Do a liver cleanse.
• Do a parasite cleanse.
• Take magnesium.
• Take melatonin.
• Take valerian root or drink valerian root tea.
• Take kava kava.
• Adjust your sleep/rise schedule. Get up at 6 a.m., retire at 10 p.m. and keep the schedule consistent, even on weekends. |

Irritable Bowel Syndrome (IBS)

A functional gastrointestinal disorder with symptoms associated with changes in how the gastrointestinal tract functions. It's not the same as colitis. In IBS the structure of the bowel is not abnormal, but it typically includes chronic abdominal discomfort.

Main Cause	Natural Cures
Several factors contribute to IBS, including stress, taking antibiotics, bacterial overgrowth, Candida, nonprescription drugs, and for some people, a disruption in the way the brain and digestive system interact.	• Do a colon cleanse. • Do a Candida cleanse. • Take probiotics. • Eat probiotic foods such as kimchi, organic plain yogurt, sauerkraut, and miso. • That omegas-3s. • Take digestive enzymes. • Drink aloe vera juice, 2 to 4 ounces at a time.

Kidney Stones

Hard masses formed in the kidneys made up of tiny crystals, typically formed by calcium compounds.

Main Cause	Natural Cures
Kidneys stones are often the result of lifestyle choices, most commonly neglecting to drink enough water. The lack of water results in an acidic environment in the	• If you have stones, consider the following: drink one gallon of distilled water combined with the juice of five organic lemons and two cups of apple cider vinegar every day for two weeks. • Do a colon cleanse.

kidneys, (too much uric acid) putting one at risk for the development of the stones. Fluoride in drinking water can lead to some types of stones. Some prescription and nonprescription medications can cause kidney stones. Being overweight increases one's risk. Recently it's been discussed that eating raw leafy greens and other vegetables can contribute to the formation of kidney stones because of their high oxalate content. Cooking removes a small percentage of oxalates. If you're getting enough water, there's little need to be too concerned about the oxalates from leafy greens unless you're consuming excessive amounts, or you've been diagnosed with a condition requiring the restriction of oxalates.

- Do a liver/gallbladder cleanse.
- Do a kidney/bladder cleanse.
- Do a parasite cleanse.
- For prevention:
- Drink plenty of pure water. Not tap water, which may be fluoridated. Drink 8 to 10 glasses a day of pure or distilled water.
- Eliminate sugar. Sugar can disrupt calcium and magnesium absorption.
- Eliminate all sodas. Sodas block calcium absorption and calcium deficiency can contribute to kidney stones.
- Eat calcium-rich foods. Calcium *supplements* can lead to stones, but eating calcium-rich foods helps prevent them. Plain, organic yogurt, sardines, wild salmon, and soy are some good choices.

Liver Problems

Liver diseases can include cirrhosis, fatty liver, jaundice, and hepatitis. Cirrhosis is when normal liver cells are replaced with scar tissue. Fatty liver is the accumulation of certain fats in the liver. Jaundice is an excess of bilirubin in the blood, usually due to obstruction of the bile duct. Hepatitis is inflammation of the liver.

Main Cause	Natural Cures
Cirrhosis: the end result of chronic liver disease. *Fatty liver*: obesity, diabetes, and poor diet. *Jaundice*: too much bilirubin (formed by the breakdown of dead red blood cells in the liver).	If you have a liver condition, see a licensed healthcare professional. A naturopathic doctor can evaluate you and come up with the right plan to restore your liver. Some suggestions: • Manage your weight. Obesity can result in fatty liver. • Do not smoke.

Hepatitis: a viral infection.	• Do a colon cleanse.
The following can lead to different types of liver problems: nonprescription drugs, prescription drugs (cholesterol reducing drugs in particular), Candida, parasites, and trans fats (hydrogenated oils).	• Do a liver/gallbladder cleanse.
	• Do a Candida cleanse.
	• Do a heavy metal cleanse.
	• Do a parasite cleanse.
	• Reduce salt intake.
	• Eliminate processed foods.
	• Eliminate excessive alcohol.
	• Eliminate prescription and nonprescription drugs.
	• If you're taking vitamin A, be sure that you're not taking too much. Excessive vitamin A is toxic to the liver.
	• Exercise to burn fat.

Lupus

An autoimmune disease where the body's immune system becomes hyperactive and begins to attack normal healthy tissue resulting in chronic inflammation and damage to skin, joints, kidneys, the blood, heart, and lungs.

Main Cause	Natural Cures
The cause of lupus is unknown. Hormones, genetics, and environmental factors are all possible contributors to the condition.	See a naturopathic doctor. With treatment, remission can be achieved.
	Doing all of the things in chapter 6 will suppress the condition.
	Some suggestions:
	• Consider taking DHEA, however, do so only with the guidance of a licensed healthcare practitioner.
	• Practice stress reduction.
	• Hypnosis has been shown to help people with the stress from lupus.
	• Exercise regularly.
	• Get adequate sleep.
	• Take omega-3s.

Male Erectile Dysfunction

A condition wherein a man is unable to get or maintain an erection firm enough to have intercourse.

Main Cause	Natural Cures
There are a number of things that can cause erectile dysfunction, including mental and emotional stress, poor circulation, nonprescription and prescription drugs, vaccines, vitamin E deficiency, calcium deficiency, diabetes, hormonal imbalance, Candida, heavy metal toxicity, and prostate problems.	• Address diabetes as discussed under the diabetes section. • Get intravenous chelation (via a licensed healthcare practitioner). • Take oral chelation—increases blood flow. • Get regular exercise. • Practice stress reduction. • Take nattokinase (for circulation). • Take natural vitamin E. • Take omega-3s. • Take ginseng. • Take Peruvian maca root. • Consider the following herbs: horny goat weed, muira puama, tribulus terrestris, gingko biloba. • Do a Candida cleanse. • Do a heavy metal cleanse.

Melanoma

A tumor of melanin forming cells that is typically cancerous.

Main Cause	Natural Cures
There is debate over the cause of melanoma. Many in the medical community say that it's due to exposure to the sun, however, that is not conclusive, as some melanomas occur in parts of the body that receive little or no sun exposure. The causes of disease are: (1) Toxins in the body. (2) Nutritional deficiencies. (3) Electromagnetic chaos. And (4) Emotional and mental stress.	• See a licensed healthcare practitioner. • Do the things in chapter 6. • Use eggplant extract cream. • Take fish oil containing vitamin D. • Eat garlic or take garlic as a supplement. • Drink green tea. • Take magnesium. • Take vitamin C. • Take vitamin D. • Take vitamin E.

One or more of those must be present to cause melanoma. Toxins in the body are one likely cause. Many types of sunscreens contain toxins and may contribute to melanoma. There are other kinds of lotions, creams, soaps, etc. people use that could contribute to melanoma. Some people may be more genetically susceptible to developing melanoma.

Migraine Headaches

Migraines are throbbing headaches that typically appear on one side of the head and are often accompanied by nausea and sensitivity to light.

Main Cause	Natural Cures
A number of things can cause migraines, including dehydration, stress, hormonal imbalance, Candida, food allergies, parasites, heavy metal toxicity, environmental allergies, and TMJ (temporomandibular joint and muscle disorders).	• Do all of the cleanses recommended in chapter 6. • Take organic apple cider vinegar (2 tablespoons in 8 ounces of pure water before meals). • Eliminate artificial sweeteners. • Practice stress reduction. • Get cranial sacral therapy. • See a chiropractor for adjustments.

Multiple Sclerosis (MS)

A chronic and typically progressive autoimmune disease that affects the brain and spinal cord.

Main Cause	Natural Cures
Heavy metal toxicity, aspartame, mental and emotional stress, viral infections, and Candida are among the factors that can cause MS.	• Do all of the things in chapter 6. • See a naturopathic doctor. • Eliminate ALL metal dental work. There have been many reports wherein removing the metal in a person's mouth has resulted in a reversal of MS. • Do a heavy metal cleanse. • Eliminate all artificial sweeteners.

	• Eliminate monosodium glutamate (MSG).
	• Use a magnetic mattress pad.
	• Do a liver/gallbladder cleanse.
	• Get alphabiotic treatments.
	• Change diet to eliminate processed foods, grains, starches, and sugar. Replace with organic foods, raw foods, and increase consumption of organic leafy greens, sulfur-rich organic vegetables (onions, broccoli, mushrooms), and bright colored organic fruits like berries. Consume wild fish high in omega-3s.
	• Improve vitamin D levels with supplement and sun exposure.

Obesity

The state of having too much body fat. An adult with a body mass index (BMI) of 30 or greater is considered obese.

Main Cause	Natural Cures
Many factors contribute to obesity, including low metabolism, mental and emotional stress, inactivity, Candida, hypoactive thyroid, inefficient pancreas, processed foods, and chemical additives in food.	• Eliminate processed foods. Anything in a box, can, or package from a major supermarket chain is likely to be processed which means it contains chemical additives. Switch to organic foods and shop in a health food store or store that contains non-processed, non-GMO food.
	• Never eat in fast food restaurants. It is not the calories and fat content that causes obesity, it is the chemical additives.
	• Do a juice fast—with guidance of a licensed healthcare practitioner.
	• Eat more raw foods and consider going for periods of time where you eat raw food exclusively.
	• Eliminate processed sugar and high fructose corn syrup. Read food labels, because high fructose corn syrup is in many foods that you might not suspect.
	• Do a colon cleanse.
	• Do a liver/gallbladder cleanse.

	• Do a parasite cleanse.
	• Do a Candida cleanse.
	• Do a heavy metal cleanse.
	• Take oral chelation.
	• Walk for an hour daily.
	• Drink at least 8 glasses of pure water daily.
	• Use extra virgin coconut oil in place of other cooking oils.
	• Take raw, organic apple cider vinegar, 2 to 4 tablespoons in 8 ounces of pure water before meals.
	• Take digestive enzymes.
	• Take probiotics.
	• Drink aloe vera juice, 2 to 4 ounces on an empty stomach.
	• Eat a balanced breakfast daily.
	• Get on a regular sleep schedule, close to rising at 6 a.m. and going to bed at 10 p.m.

Phobias

Extreme fear of, or aversion to something.

Main Cause	Natural Cures
A definitive cause of phobias is unknown and they are unique to each individual, however some phobias may run in families or have cultural connections. Phobias usually begin in childhood and can be the result of traumatic experiences. Recent studies have revealed that fears and phobias can be passed to subsequent generations via DNA, which means they can be inherited.	• If you suffer from a phobia consider hypnosis. Hypnosis reprograms the subconscious and has been shown to be a successful treatment for phobias.
	• Look into Callahan Thought Field Therapy (TFT) techniques. Tapping and TFT were developed by Robert Callahan. You can find TFT practitioners around the country via an online search. Many people find relief from all kinds of issues via tapping.
	• Consider Emotional Freedom Technique (EFT)—As with TFT, you may find EFT practitioners in various parts of the country via an online search. Gary Craig was a student of Robert Callahan and developed EFT.

PMS
Period prior to menstrual cycle wherein uncomfortable symptoms arise, including bloating, breast tenderness, food cravings, fatigue, sadness, tension, irritability, and mood swings.

Main Cause	Natural Cures
Calcium and magnesium deficiency, hormonal imbalance, thyroid abnormality, heavy metal toxicity, Candida, nonprescription and prescription drugs, mental and emotional stress.	• A change in diet may help PMS symptoms. Reduce sugar and caffeine. Eat raw organic fruits and vegetables. Drink fresh organic juices. • Take calcium and magnesium supplements. • Do a colon cleanse. • Do a liver/gallbladder cleanse. • Do a heavy metal cleanse. • Do a parasite cleanse. • Use stress reduction techniques—deep breathing, yoga, meditation. • Eat and/or cook with extra virgin coconut oil—helps with hormones.

Peripheral Vascular Disease
A condition of the blood vessels that can lead to narrowing and ultimately hardening of the arteries.

Main Cause	Natural Cures
Plaque buildup in the arteries, smoking, high cholesterol, obesity, and diabetes contribute to peripheral vascular disease.	• See a licensed healthcare practitioner. • If you're overweight, lose weight. • Quit smoking. • Walk regularly, preferably daily. This stimulates the opening of blood vessels in lower legs. (Symptoms of this condition include lower leg pain.) • Take vitamin C—helps with inflammation and keeps lining of arteries strong. • Take vitamin E—helps thin the blood. • Take and/or eat garlic—helps thin the blood. • Take ginkgo biloba—enhances blood flow. • Take oral chelation.

Snoring
Hoarse or harsh breathing sound during sleep.

Main Cause	Natural Cures
Dehydration, Candida, excess weight (which puts pressure on airways), blockage in the nose resulting from a deformed nasal septum, nasal polyps, allergies, sleeping pills, antihistamines, and alcohol consumed close to bedtime may all cause snoring.	• Use essential oil throat spray. • Change sleeping position. Sleeping on the back promotes snoring. Try sleeping on the side. • If overweight, losing weight can help. • Avoid alcohol, especially within 4 hours of going to sleep. • Open nasal passages either with steam from a hot shower or with "Breathe right" strips.

Sore Throat
Painful inflammation of the pharynx.

Main Cause	Natural Cures
Bacterial and viral infections cause sore throats. Candida and parasites are other possible causes to consider.	If a sore throat continues for more than a few days, see a licensed healthcare practitioner because the condition could be the result of a more serious illness. Some suggestions: • Gargle with colloidal silver or colloidal minerals. • Gargle with Himalayan pink sea salt and warm purified water. • Gargle with goldenseal root powder and warm purified water. • Mix coconut oil (1 tablespoon) with raw honey (1 teaspoon) and 2 tablespoons of organic lemon juice. Heat if necessary. Sip slowly and let the mixture coat the throat. All three ingredients are antibacterial and will help heal the inflammation. • Do a Candida cleanse. • Do a parasite cleanse. • Do a heavy metal cleanse. • Take the herbs cat's claw and larrea.

Tumors
An abnormal growth of body tissue.

Main Cause	Natural Cures
Toxic overload, electromagnetic chaos such as cell phones or laptop computers, mental and emotional stress, Candida, and viral infections are causes of tumors.	• Do all of the things in chapter 6, particularly the cleanses. • See a licensed healthcare practitioner. Some suggestions: • Take food grade hydrogen peroxide therapy (35%). • Get ozone therapy. • Take oral and/or intravenous chelation therapy. • Take flaxseed oil. • Take shark cartilage. • Use infrared saunas. • Practice stress reduction. • Get energetic rebalancing (AIM program, www.AIMprogram.com).

Varicose Veins
Varicose veins are veins that have become enlarged due to being filled with an abnormal collection of blood.

Main Cause	Natural Cures
Nonprescription and prescription drugs, mental and emotional stress, trans fats, homogenized dairy products, vitamin E deficiency, and being overweight contribute to varicose veins.	• See an herbalist who can prescribe an herbal remedy specifically for you. • Some herbs to consider are horse chestnut extract, grape seed extract, and butcher's broom, all of which have been shown to be helpful in eliminating varicose veins. Some suggestions: • Take natural vitamin E. • Take omega-3s. • Take nattokinase. • Take oral chelation and/or intravenous chelation.

It's important to understand that while specific cures are excellent information to have, they're only *one part* of what needs to be done to restore the body to health. The conditions I've covered above can and should be addressed by implementing the things in chapter 6. It's important to know that people who are looking for a "specific cure" for a "specific disease" are completely missing the point of this book. You must undergo an entire lifestyle change in order to be fully cured and that's why you must absorb this book in its entirety, not just this chapter.

> You must undergo an entire lifestyle change in order to be fully cured...

A disease is nothing more than a label put on a series of symptoms. The symptoms could be caused by hundreds of factors, or combinations of factors. This is one of the things that medical science does not want you to know about. In order for the medical community to make money, they must "isolate" a specific something so they can find a drug that can be patented to treat it. The medical community would prescribe that one expensive drug to treat the symptoms of all kinds of people without understanding each individual's *cause* for developing those symptoms. If you were to take a hundred people who were experiencing the exact same symptom, a migraine headache for example, each person's migraine headache could have a different cause. This means every person's treatment should be different. What will work for one person might not work for another.

This is why when you ask, "What's the cure for X?" the answer is I don't know, because no one knows until you're looked at by a healthcare practitioner, analyzed, and the cause is determined. Once the cause is determined, then the right treatment will be discussed. For example, if you have genital herpes, we all know the cause is a virus. What we don't know is why the virus became active in you. Everyone gets exposed to the virus, but not everyone develops breakouts and succumbs to it. So even though we do know that it's a virus, if you had five people with a genital herpes breakout, each person's reason for succumbing to the herpes virus could be different; therefore, the treatment that would work for each of the five people could be slightly different. In one person red marine algae may completely kill the virus and he or she would never have an outbreak again. In another person it could be the herb larrea; in another person hydrogen peroxide applied to the breakout could kill the virus; in another person dimethyl sulfoxide (DMSO) applied to the breakout area could kill the virus; in another person lysine could suppress the symptoms. In some people, they may need to use a combination of treatments. This is why individualized treatment is necessary.

When you look at a hundred sick people with different illnesses, you do find some common denominators. Most sick people are dehydrated; most sick people need a colon cleanse; most sick people need a liver/gallbladder cleanse; most sick people have a Candida yeast overgrowth; most sick people have parasites; most sick people have nutritional deficiencies; most sick people's bodies are loaded with toxins; most sick people have some type of emotional or mental stress that has been trapped in their physical body; most sick people have heavy metal toxicities; most sick people have environmental and food allergies and don't even realize it. This is why I always tell people who have any physical problems to do the things in chapter 6, and then reevaluate their condition in three to six months. It is amazing that the majority of people see their symptoms diminish dramatically, or even vanish.

A few years ago, I received a call from a seventy-eight year old woman who told me she'd been on five different prescription drugs for over ten years. Her symptoms continually got worse. Then she read my book and started implementing the things in chapter 6. She did this under the care of a licensed healthcare practitioner who didn't use drugs and surgery. Within three months she got completely off of all her prescription medications, and told me that she did about half of the recommendations in chapter 6. She said she felt twenty-five years younger and full of energy, full of vitality, and all of her symptoms and conditions were cured.

This is not an isolated incident. I'm constantly hearing stories from people who read the first version of this book and implemented the cures.

Larry said, "I was on a number of medications—anti-depressants, acid reflux medication, I had high blood pressure, high cholesterol, arthritis, I was forty to fifty pounds overweight, always tired, and had no energy. I read *Natural Cures*. Now I don't go to the doctor and I don't get sick. I don't have acid reflux, I don't have high cholesterol, I don't have high blood pressure, I don't have gout or arthritis anymore. I am drug free."

Dan said, "Before I read the book, I was diagnosed with incurable cancer. Stage 3B melanoma. Didn't have a good prognosis— less than a 2% chance survival rate. With that type of cancer, chemo and radiation weren't options. So I was really looking into some recommendations for treatments. I mentioned to my doctors that I'd hold off on the surgery and try some things on my own. They told me I was making a big mistake. 'There's no proof that's going to help and you'll waste a lot of money. ' So I said, 'Well, wish me luck anyways. I'm going to check it out.' So we started eating organic and started to detox and we jumped in. A four year journey, full-time, did some crazy things, and in the end, I'm cancer free."

Julianne said, "*Natural Cures* saved my life. I had a genetically passed down heart condition, and the doctors one day looked at me and said, 'You have about a month to live.' I was around fifteen, sixteen years old. I had no awareness that the food I was eating had GMOs and was literally destroying my body at such a young age. I picked up the book, my mom had it, and was able to change my diet, change the way I was living my life and within months, my heart was strong."

These kind of "miraculous " cures continue to happen to thousands of people all over the world every week. It could happen for you.

> ...if you're sick, you must see a licensed healthcare practitioner who does not use only drugs and surgery.

Let me emphasize again, if you're sick, you must see a licensed healthcare practitioner who does not use only drugs and surgery. In my opinion, you must be on an energetic rebalancing program. You must do a colon cleanse, a liver/gallbladder cleanse, a kidney/bladder cleanse, a Candida cleanse, a parasite cleanse, a heavy metal cleanse, and, ideally, a full-body cleanse. You must stop all nonprescription and prescription drugs. You must stop eating poisons such as fast food and artificial sweeteners. You must be drinking at least eight to ten glasses of purified water every day. You must use some technology to eliminate the stress your body is holding on to. If you don't do these basic things, it's impossible, in my opinion, for you to truly get your body back in a state of balance, eliminate your symptoms, and cure yourself of disease.

To return to good health, the most important thing you can do is take personal responsibility and decide that you *are* going to find the cause and cure for your disease. In order to do this, in my opinion, you must seek out licensed healthcare practitioners to assist you. Please do not attempt to treat yourself without guidance from a professional. Though I have copious knowledge about the causes, cures, and prevention of disease, I still seek the advice and opinions of licensed healthcare practitioners regularly. I do this to prevent disease, gain knowledge, and to get other people's perspectives. I don't believe I'm the smartest guy in the world. And I believe that two heads are better than one. If you truly want to prevent and/ or cure disease, it's vital that you seek advice. That said, it's equally important that you not look at these people as "all-knowing gods." Get several opinions and understand that what you're getting are just that—*opinions*. You must gather the information yourself, listen to the various points of view, review them, and decide the course of action that *you* feel is most beneficial. Remember, it's your body, your health, and your life. You take responsibility.

To find a licensed healthcare practitioner you can go to your local Yellow Pages (if you still use it), or do an online search. I recommend that you start with a naturopathic doctor (N.D.). An N.D. is highly trained and able to treat a wide variety of health problems. An N.D. will also be able to direct you to other health-care professionals that are appropriate for your situation. These may include chiropractors, massage therapists, colon therapists, herbalists, etc. You can do your own online searches for any of those and also for other modalities in the "natural healthcare arena" such as oriental medicine, homeopathy, acupuncture, iridology, holistic medicine etc. But if you begin with being evaluated by a naturopathic doctor, he or she will likely be helpful in advising what treatments will be useful to you. Even if you're not sick, or experiencing any negative symptoms, I encourage you to visit a variety of licensed healthcare practitioners now, for the maintenance of optimum health. Better to *prevent* disease than to worry about trying to cure it once you have it.

CHAPTER 12

Frequently Asked Questions

Since this book was published, millions of people have been exposed to the fact that: (a) drugs and surgery are ineffective and cause most diseases, (b) the food produced by the publicly traded food corporations and fast food restaurants causes illness and disease, and (c) there are natural non-drug and nonsurgical ways to prevent and cure virtually every disease. Because of the success of this book, many health advocates who promote organic food and health experts who promote non-drug and nonsurgical ways to prevent and cure disease, are now becoming more mainstream. With so many voices talking about the subject, there are obviously different opinions regarding natural remedies. This is good. As I mentioned early on, nobody has a monopoly on the truth, including me. There are no such things as "facts," there are only *opinions* based on the information we currently have. Health experts may therefore come up with slightly different perspectives on what a person should do for his or her best health outcome.

That said, I'd like to address some of the most frequently asked questions I receive regarding health and nutrition, and the concepts covered in this book. Even if you don't think a question is relevant to you, please keep reading, because the answer may be more relevant than you thought.

Question: My doctor says I need drugs and/or surgery. What do I do?

Answer: First, I would encourage you to stop going to medical doctors who only prescribe drugs and surgery. I'd encourage you to also get advice from licensed healthcare practitioners who don't prescribe drugs and surgery. Get three or four opinions. This way you can make an informed decision. Your condition may be past the point of no return, where only drugs and surgery would be effective in keeping you alive a little longer. However, I believe that anyone who says that you "need" drugs and surgery is either misinformed, not knowledgeable about natural methods, or simply trying to make money on your illness.

Question: Can I ever eat a cheeseburger again, or go to a fast food restaurant?

Answer: You can eat cheeseburgers and French fries as long as you make them at home with organic ingredients. People always ask me what I eat. I eat anything and everything (with some exceptions) as long as it's certified organic. You can eat beef, cheese, butter, milk, cream, eggs, lamb, chicken, duck, mashed potatoes, French fries, onion rings, ice cream, chocolate, you name it, as long as it's organic. No, you cannot eat in fast food restaurants if you want to cure yourself of disease and remain healthy. Fast food restaurants use chemical ingredients to grow, process, and manufacture their so-called food. The chemicals, the lack of nutrients and the outrageous number of free radicals in their energetically altered food is making you sick.

Question: So, is fast food really that bad?

Answer: Yes. Fast food absolutely causes illness and disease, including cancer, diabetes, and a host of other major health problems. Fast food makes you fat. Fast food is purposely produced with chemical additives that are designed to increase your appetite, get you physically and chemically addicted, and make you fat. The fast food industry is knowingly causing illness and disease. McDonald's itself stated that it's a matter of common knowledge that any processing that its foods undergo serve to make them more harmful than unprocessed foods. An example is McNuggets. These were originally made from old chickens that could no longer lay eggs. Now they're made from chickens that have unusually large breasts, a kind of genetically altered and produced animal. The manufacturing process includes stripping the meat from the bone and grinding it up in a mash. It is then combined with a host of preservatives, stabilizers, and other chemicals, pressed into shapes, breaded, deep fried, freeze-dried, and then shipped to McDonald's. Judge Robert Sweet called them "a McFrankenstein creation of various elements not utilized by the home cook."

I encourage you to view the documentary *Supersize Me*, which is available on DVD. This is a must watch for anyone who eats at fast food restaurants. This film examines the **question:** *What if a person ate nothing but McDonald's food for thirty days?* Could thirty days of eating nothing but McDonald's cause medical problems? Could just thirty days of eating McDonald's food cause massive weight gain? Could thirty days of eating McDonald's food cause disease and illness? This documentary shows the truth. The man had his blood work tested before, during, and after his experiment. He had his weight checked. In just thirty days, the medical doctors were astonished by what happened to his body. In just thirty days of eating McDonald's food he gained twenty-five pounds. No doctor could believe it. I can believe it because I know that McDonald's, like every other fast food restaurant, in my opinion, is purposely putting ingredients in the food to get you physically addicted to it, to increase your appetite, and make you fat. This movie certainly substantiates this opinion. From a health standpoint, the doctors were shocked that his liver virtually turned to fat and his cholesterol shot up sixty-five points. His body-fat percentage went from 11 percent to over 18 percent. He nearly doubled his risk of coronary heart disease. He said he felt depressed and exhausted most of the time. His moods swung on a dime, and his sex life suffered. He craved McDonald's food, and got headaches when he didn't eat it. The doctor said if he stayed on this diet, he would develop coronary artery disease, inflammation, hardening of the liver, and probably develop dozens of other illnesses and die an early death.

The doctors who did his blood work could not believe how he was, in effect, *dying* after just thirty days. They couldn't believe it because they were only looking at calories, carbohydrates, protein, fat, and sodium. They weren't considering the "trans fats." They weren't considering how the food has been genetically produced. They weren't considering how the food was energetically destroyed and toxic. They weren't considering all of the food processing chemicals and additives. That's the reason this man became so sick in such a short time. This is why you need to know that if you're sick and you're eating fast food, or food from publicly traded corporations, they are in fact making you sick. It is the poisons, chemicals, additives, and energetic altering of the food that's making you ill.

Fast food restaurants, like all food manufacturers, have one objective and that is to increase profits. They increase profits by getting more of your money. One of the ways they get you to buy more food is by increasing the portion size.

When French fries were first sold at McDonald's there was one size. That size French fries is now the "small." McDonald's also has a medium, a large, and a super-size. The original size is still there, but few people order it. The difference is the original size is 200 calories, but the super-size is over 600 calories.

When Burger King first opened they sold a twelve-ounce small soda and a sixteen-ounce large soda. Today, the twelve-ounce soda is called "kiddy" size, the sixteen-ounce is no longer a large; it's now the "small." They have a medium, which is thirty-two ounces, and a forty-two ounce size. This is pretty much across the board at all fast food restaurants.

In 2013, New York City's then Mayor Bloomberg tried to ban these outrageously large sodas, however, the ban was struck down as a violation of principle of "separation of powers." In *Supersize Me* it was mentioned that cars have introduced larger cup holders to accommodate those huge 7-Eleven double gulps, which are sixty-four ounces, a full half gallon, and hold anywhere from six-hundred to eight-hundred calories. Just imagine, a half gallon of soda for one person. That's forty-eight teaspoons of sugar!

Fast food restaurants also are involved in some of the most devious advertising campaigns ever. This is similar to what happened in the tobacco industry. As discussed in *Supersize Me*, a secret study by one of the tobacco companies was about brand imprinting for later acquisition in life. What this means is the tobacco companies would produce things such as toy cigarettes, so that a child at age four, five, or six would "play smoke" them. The theory was that even though the little child had no understanding of what they were doing, they were imprinting their memory with the act of smoking. So when they grew to the age where they were allowed to smoke, without realizing it, they would be going for that pack and recognize it because they had those nice feelings when they were a kid.

The same goes for children at the playgrounds at fast food restaurants like McDonald's and Burger King. They bring the children in, they have fun, they have warm fuzzy feelings, and later in life they relive those feelings when they go to their fast food restaurant. This is being done purposely by the fast food industry to increase sales down the road. You have to understand, the fast food industry is spending millions of dollars researching ways to get people hooked on their products. Kids who eat in fast food restaurants as little as three times a week have elevated abnormal liver function tests. Under a microscope there is evidence of scarring of the liver, fibrosis of the liver, and early states of sclerosis. This is all caused by fast food.

In addition to viewing *Supersize Me,* I also encourage you to read the book *Fast Food Nation* and or watch the film of the same name so you can see just how bad fast food really is, not only for your health, but for society in general. Think about this: The average American child sees ten-thousand food advertisements per year on TV alone. Ninety-five percent of those are for sugared cereals, soft drinks, fast food, and candy. It's not a fair fight. The food industry has the money to brainwash children into buying their products. Sadly, when children are shown pictures of people like George Washington, Abraham Lincoln, and Jesus Christ, they often have no idea who these people are. But when they're shown a picture of Ronald McDonald, every single one knows his name. And what's even sadder is they believe that he's a "good man" who's helping children. This is how the food industry misleads and brainwashes our kids.

Think about this, as discussed in the movie *Supersize Me,* companies spend billions of dollars making sure you know about their product. In 2001, on direct media advertising alone (radio, television, and print) McDonald's spent $1.4 billion worldwide getting you to buy their products. On direct media advertising Pepsi spent more than $1 billion. To advertise its candy, Hershey Foods spent almost $200 million. In its peak year, the five-a-day fruit and vegetable campaign had a total advertising budget, in *all* media, of just $2 million. That's a hundred times less than the direct media budget of one food company. We're being bombarded by the food industry with lies and deceptions that brainwash us into believing that their products are healthy for us, and it's working. Think about the way food is marketed: T-shirts, coupons, toys for children, giveaways in fast food places, etc. The most heavily advertised foods are the most consumed. That's no surprise. Whoever spends the most money on advertising sells the most food.

> All fast food companies and junk food manufacturers want you to be physically addicted to their food...

Think about this scary fact—the majority of people tested could not recite the "Pledge of Allegiance," however almost all of them could sing the Big Mac song, "Two all-beef patties, special sauce, lettuce, cheese, pickles, onions on a sesame seed bun." You're probably singing it right now.

One of the scariest things is how fast food is being sold in schools. When you look at the school lunch programs, the most appalling observation is about junk food companies that make huge profits off of the schools. Junk food companies don't want to get kicked out of the school system. They want to be there to addict the children so they'll have them as customers for life. This points out that food manufacturers know their foods are dangerous and cause harm to the body. They don't care. They specifically target children, demanding that soda machines and junk food be sold in schools, which guarantees that these kids will have illness and disease, because as publicly traded corporations they have one objective: To increase profits. Therefore, they'll do anything, hurt anyone, and destroy people's lives by giving them disease, all in the name of making more money.

All fast food companies and junk food manufacturers want you to be physically addicted to their food, just like drug dealers want you to become physically addicted to their drugs. This is why these companies have spent millions in secret laboratories producing chemical additives that get you physically addicted to the food, increase your appetite, and make you fat. The chemical-laden products that McDonald's and other fast food companies sell are essentially drugs. Internal documents at McDonald's refer to the people who eat their food at least once a week as "heavy users." Seventy-two percent of people who eat at McDonald's are heavy users. They also have another category, the "super heavy user." These people eat their food three, four, five times a week and up. Twenty-two percent of the people who eat at McDonald's are super heavy users. *Supersize Me* states that if you look at the menu at a fast food restaurant they use all of the addicting components. They'll take a slab of meat, cover it with cheese, and then serve it with a sugary soda, which has the addictive powers of sugar with plenty of added caffeine. Give this to a twelve year old and his or her brain is no match for that chemical combination.

I wondered about the health of the 22 percent of people who ate at McDonald's three, four, five times a week and up. In my observations, I found that these people are riddled with disease. I found that people who eat at McDonald's three times a week or more have the highest chance of getting cancer, diabetes, obesity, heart disease, acid reflux, constipation, sleep disorders, depression, eczema, dandruff, and a host of other medical disorders. McDonald's will, of course, disagree with my observations. In my opinion, they are the new "evil empire." Remember, the food industry uses lobbyists in Washington to make sure that no government agency ever says *eat less* of its products, and to make sure that the government never passes legislation that could hurt the industry's profits.

So the bottom line answer to the question is absolutely *never* eat in a fast food restaurant.

Question: Why don't you talk about calories, fats, protein, or carbohydrates?

Answer: While those things are important, they're not as important to discuss as the chemicals and poisons put into our food supply. The chemical fertilizers and the pesticides used in the food, the fact that the food is picked too early and then gassed, and the fact that the food is genetically modified and manufactured in natural ways is far more important than the number of calories, or the fat and carbohydrate content, because the unnatural, chemical-laden food will make you hungry, addicted, and fat. That's what everyone is missing.

Question: How are you qualified to write this book when you're not a medical doctor?

Answer: The number one qualification I have to write this book is precisely the fact that I am not a medical doctor. If I were a medical doctor, I'd be unqualified to write it. Think about it. If you're a medical doctor, you spent the majority of your training on traditional medical practices, including prescribing drugs and surgery. How can you wake up one day and say that everything you've been taught is wrong; everything that was drilled into your head, that you were forced to believe, is false? It would be next to impossible. How can medical doctors be qualified to talk about health and nutrition when they have little to no training in natural methods of prevention and curing disease?

My qualifications are that I'm logical, I use common sense, and I can see the truth. I've also done extensive research, traveled around the world, interviewed thousands of patients and doctors, been treated by hundreds of licensed alternative healthcare practitioners, studied volumes of books, research papers, and other documents; and I've made billions of dollars in business, which has put me in corporate boardrooms all around the world dealing with the most powerful people on the planet. I know the inner workings of government and of corporations, and I know the greed. I also know about the insatiable appetite to make money at all costs. I know about the fraud and deception that goes on behind closed doors. I've been a part of it, such a part of it that I spent two years in federal prison. I understand more about the inner workings of the moneymaking machines and political machines around the world than most people. I also live everything I talk about. I've experienced it and I've seen the results in my friends, my family, and myself. Plus, I'm 156 years old and have virtually never been sick. (Just kidding!)

Question: How come I never hear about the stuff you say on the radio or on TV, and I never see it in newspapers and magazines?

Answer: As I've mentioned, newspapers, magazines, radio, and television are outlets owned by publicly traded corporations whose main interest is in making a profit, not in providing truthful information. They'll produce stories that get the best ratings, because good ratings mean good profits. Unfortunately, the sponsors of these media outlets (the advertisers) also control the message you hear on television and radio, and read in newspapers and magazines. And since the majority of advertisers are pharmaceutical companies and major food companies, you're never going to get the truth that the food industry and pharmaceutical industry are making you ill.

Question: Is there a difference between fitness and health?

Answer: Absolutely. A person can be exceptionally fit, yet also unhealthy. Jim Fixx was a well-known runner who wrote *The Complete Book of Running*. He dropped dead of a heart attack at age 52 after inspiring many people to become fit. He ran daily, and appeared to be very fit, but his arteries had blockages and he was *not* healthy. There are other people who may be slightly overweight, and they may not be strong or flexible, yet they're very healthy and may even live to be a hundred years old. Generally speaking, there's a balance between fitness and health. In order to be super healthy you have to be at least moderately fit; but you can be exceptionally fit and still develop diseases and die young. It is more important to be healthy than fit, but for those who want to look good in a bathing suit, being fit is more important. I believe in both fitness and health, but health should take priority over fitness. If health is your number one priority, your fitness level is probably going to be better than average anyway.

Question: How do I change my body pH from acid to alkaline?

Answer: Do all of the things in chapter 6.

Question: Why is a liver cleanse so important?

Answer: The liver is the only organ that can pump fat out of the body. The liver is also the filter and cleanser of the bloodstream. Most people, in my opinion, have a sluggish liver. If your liver is sluggish, you can't burn fat properly, and you can't filter and clean your blood properly. That means you're setting yourself up for illness and disease. Your liver is sluggish because of all of the chemicals and toxins in the food you eat, as well as all of the nonprescription and prescription drugs you've taken. If you're taking cholesterol-reducing drugs, you definitely have a sluggish liver. If you've ever taken an antibiotic in your life, that antibiotic has killed the friendly bacteria in your intestine, causing a Candida yeast overgrowth, which always attacks the liver. When most people do a liver cleanse, they feel so much better and can't believe the difference.

Question: Are we really full of toxins, and will doing cleanses really prevent and cure diseases as serious as cancer, diabetes, or heart disease?

Answer: Yes. Every person has toxic material in his or her body causing illness and disease. Yes, by doing a colon cleanse, a liver/

gallbladder cleanse, a kidney/ bladder cleanse, a heavy metal cleanse, a parasite cleanse, a Candida cleanse, and a full-body fat cleanse you can prevent yourself from getting sick, as well as cure yourself of even the most horrible diseases. Yes, doing the recommended cleanse is one of the "natural cures" that they don't want you to know about. Here's a questionnaire to ascertain just how toxic you are. Answer each question yes or no. If you answer yes to over twenty questions, you are highly toxic.

1. I've received vaccines.

2. I've taken antibiotics in my life.

3. I've taken prescription drugs in the last five years.

4. I've taken aspirin, Tylenol, ibuprofen, or other over-the-counter pain medication.

5. I've taken over-the-counter nonprescription drugs.

6. I shower and/or bathe in regular tap water.

7. I drink water out of the tap.

8. I have been in a swimming pool where chlorine was used.

9. I use a cellular telephone without any electromagnetic chaos protection.

10. I use a laptop computer with a wireless device.

11. I watch TV.

12. I own and watch a high-definition television.

13. I use a wireless telephone in my house.

14. I use a remote control for my television or other electronic appliances.

15. I have a satellite television.

16. I drive in a car every day.

17. I drive in heavy traffic.

18. I use hair dyes.

19. I use fingernail polish.

20. I use makeup and cosmetics.

21. I use moisturizers, body lotions, and sunscreens on my skin.

22. I use air fresheners in my house.

23. I use bug spray in my house.

24. I use standard cleaning products in my house.

25. I use standard soap and detergent for my skin and my clothes.

26. I use toothpaste with fluoride.

27. I eat in fast food restaurants at least once a month.

28. I eat in restaurants at least once a month.

29. I eat products produced by large publicly traded corporations.

30. I buy brand name food products that are heavily advertised on TV.

31. I eat food that is not certified 100 percent organic.

32. I eat beef, lamb, poultry, eggs, and dairy products that are not organic.

33. I eat pork and shellfish.

34. I use artificial sweeteners such as NutraSweet or Splenda.

35. I drink sodas at least several times a week.

36. I drink diet sodas at least several times a week.

37. I don't have at least one large bowel movement each day.

38. I use nonstick pans to cook with.

39. I use deodorant and antiperspirant.

40. I do not drink eight glasses of purified water every day.

41. I have never had a colonic or enema.

42. I live near high-tension power lines.

43. I live within a few miles of a manufacturing plant of some kind.

44. I live within a hundred miles of an agricultural area where produce is grown.

45. I live within a hundred miles of ranches where livestock, cattle, chickens, or other animals are raised.

This is a quick list that I hope will open your eyes to the fact that simply living a "normal life" results in a lot of toxins going into your body. Keep in mind this is a relatively new phenomena. A hundred years ago people were not exposed to so many toxins in the environment. A hundred years ago people weren't loading their bodies with huge amounts of toxins the way we are today. Every single year the level of toxins we're exposed to increases. The level of toxins in the air, in the water supply, and the food supply are constantly rising. The level of toxins surrounding our environment and our living spaces are rising. The level of electromagnetic chaos is increasing. The amount of nonprescription and prescription drugs is going up. The amount of chemicals used in the production of our food is going up. The amount of toxins being force-fed to us by large publicly traded corporations continues to rise. So yes, you are absolutely toxic, and yes, by cleaning the toxins out of your body you *can* produce miraculous cures.

Question: Can we really get disease just by breathing the air?

Answer: Sadly, yes we can. The *Associated Press* reports that toxic dust is a household threat. The article states that Americans are exposed to a variety of potentially dangerous chemicals in their homes from products such as computers, frying pans, shower curtains, cleaning chemicals, bug sprays, etc. A study found thirty-five hazardous industrial chemicals in household dust samples. This brings home the fact that hazardous chemicals are in our daily lives. All of these chemicals are known to be harmful to the immune, respiratory, cardiovascular, and reproductive systems. Infants and children are especially vulnerable. The lobbying group, the American Chemistry Council, which represents major chemical companies, made the insane statement: "Just because a toxic substance is found in dust or in the body doesn't necessarily mean it causes health problems." This is why you need air filters and air cleaners and you must start using nontoxic, organic cleaning products in your home.

Question: Are all brand named popular foods sold by publicly traded corporations bad?

Answer: Yes. Remember, natural food, organic food, is fine. It's when the profit motive becomes the main objective that those foods stop being natural and are in effect manufactured. This is when the situation causes obesity and disease. Think about the average farmer. He wants to produce some vegetables and make a profit. The problem is chemical companies bombard him with sales pitches telling "Farmer Joe" how he can increase his yield and increase his profits by using their fantastic chemicals. So Farmer Joe buys genetically modified seed that he's told will produce more crops faster and also be germ resistant. Farmer Joe also uses chemical fertilizers to make the vegetables grow at an unnaturally, unhealthy fast rate. He then sprays poisonous pesticides and herbicides on his vegetables. These are all absorbed into the vegetables and cannot be washed off. In order to make the vegetables look beautiful and last longer, they are picked before they are ripe and put into a gas chamber and sprayed with more chemicals. They are then shipped to the grocery store where they can last for days or weeks without spoiling. You then eat them. The problem is that the product is genetically modified, full of toxins and chemicals, devoid of any nutrients and, because of the irradiation, energetically changed, causing the food to be toxic to the body.

Question: Can something as serious as multiple sclerosis be cured with natural methods?

Answer: Yes. A few months ago I met a woman who had multiple sclerosis. She had a cane and couldn't walk very well. She recognized me from television and asked if I was the author of the *Natural Cures* book. I said yes. She then said that she read the book and didn't understand how anything in it could help her with her multiple sclerosis. As she said this I noticed that she had a diet soda in her hand. I explained that MS, like all diseases, is caused by too many toxins in the body, nutritional deficiencies, electromagnetic chaos, and/or stress. I asked her how long she had been drinking diet soda. She said most of her life. I asked her if she had a lot of dental work. She said her mouth was filled with dental work and various kinds of metal. I told her that the majority of MS sufferers who I'd seen had experienced tremendous results by eliminating aspartame, the artificial sweetener in diet sodas, getting rid of all of the metal in their mouth, and sleeping on a magnetic mattress pad. Most also have Lyme disease, which can be cured with homeopathies, intravenous hydrogen peroxide therapy, and other natural therapies. Usually sufferers see tremendous relief in just a matter of weeks or months. She said it didn't sound like it would help, but she'd give it a try. I gave her my number and told her to call me, as I was curious about her results. I also let her know that I was not a doctor or a licensed healthcare practitioner and could not treat her, and that she must seek professional help. Three months later she called to tell me that she could not believe the spectacular results she had experienced; she said she felt like a new woman and she felt fifteen years younger. This is a good example of how simple "natural cures" work.

Question: How do I recharge after burnout?

Answer: There are several things you can do if you feel burned out or approaching that stage. For one, spend some time alone because it's important you nurture yourself to regain a sense of wellbeing and a nourished inner life. There is still some social stigma associated with spending time alone. But that is slowly eroding as new research shows the health benefits of periodic solitude. Try going to the movies by yourself, for a walk alone, or even taking a vacation on your own.

Another approach is setting new boundaries to protect yourself from becoming overwhelmed. The next time the PTA calls and says they absolutely need you at the bake sale, consider that there are likely hundreds of other parents at the school your child attends who could fill in. Particularly if you've already done your part in the past. Or, if you're called at home or emailed after work hours, wait to respond when you're back on the job.

On a lighter note, do you enjoy driving? If so, then take the long way home and use the time to crank up the radio. Sing along or just decompress. Take a walk or go to the gym. Go out for lunch with a friend, watch television or do something else that will take your mind off of the pressures of the day. Find something to laugh about. Take a vacation.

Question: Will "natural cures" work for everybody?

Answer: I believe "natural cures" will work for everyone, but the specific *natural cure* that works for one person's symptoms may not work for another. An example is not everyone who smokes cigarettes comes down with lung cancer, but 90 percent of the people who develop lung cancer smoke cigarettes. What this means is not every single person who drinks diet soda will come down with multiple sclerosis, but almost everyone who comes down with multiple sclerosis probably is adversely affected by the aspartame in the diet soda. This is an important aspect to understand. The reason for this apparent inconsistency is that everyone's genetic strengths and weaknesses are different. The four causes of all disease (too many toxins in the body, nutritional deficiencies, electromagnetic chaos, and/or stress) affect the genetically weak areas in a person. Therefore, two people could do exactly the same things and one person could come down with a disease and another person may not. This is also why two people can do the exact same "natural cure" and one person will see spectacular results and another person may not see the same exceptional results. However, there is a "natural cure" that the second person could use that would lead to great results. That is why doing the things in chapter 6 is so vitally important for prevention and curing of disease.

Closing Thoughts

Throughout this book I've repeatedly made the statement, "I'm mad as hell and I'm not going to take it anymore." Many who read this feel my outrage at the lies and deceptions perpetrated against people by our government, the FDA and the FTC, as well as large, publicly traded corporations, all in the effort to increase their power, influence, and money. I am doing this because it's a calling. I believe it's my mission to help educate people and make society a better place. I'm sincerely grateful to know that my mission is having a positive impact on millions of people's lives, while also having a negative impact on the power, influence, and profits of the "Goliaths" around the world.

I've been offered tens of millions of dollars to stop saying what I'm saying. One organization offered me $100 million dollars if I would stop my consumer advocacy work, stop blowing the whistle on insider information, and simply live a quiet life. Prominent and powerful people, who will remain nameless, have assured me that if I continue my mission I will be repeatedly sued, attacked, debunked, ridiculed, persecuted in the media, the press, and in the courts. I've been threatened in every way you can imagine.

All of these things only bolster my resolve.

I refuse to be bribed or bought. I refuse to cave in to pressure. I will not live my life operating from fear.

It's gratifying to know that the work I'm doing is having a positive impact. Every week I receive correspondence from people telling me how they're off drugs and how their symptoms and illnesses have been cured. When I listen to how people's lives have changed for the better, how they're saving money, and how the pain in their bodies is gone, I know that what I am doing is right. Every time I speak publicly or do a presentation, I close my eyes and wish for at least one person to be positively impacted by the information. That's what makes my mission worth it. I hope you are that person. I hope this book has made a difference in your life. I hope that it helps you to begin an exciting and beautiful journey. I invite you to stay updated with new natural cures through my newsletter (which you can order through my website at www.NaturalCuresBook.com/newsletter) and to share your success stories by emailing me at mystory@ NaturalCuresSuccess.com. May your family be happier, healthier, and wealthier because you apply the knowledge I've shared. We've all heard the phrase "knowledge is power," but in actuality, knowledge is only power *if* you *use* it. The knowledge you've gained will only benefit you and your family when you use it. The wonderful author Leo Buscaglia once said, "To know and not to do is not to know." Apply these techniques in your life and as I mentioned in the beginning of this book, I *know* you'll never be the same.

> ...knowledge is only power if you use it.

Humbly yours in health,

Kevin Trudeau

Resources

Websites:

Acupressure
www.acupressure.com

Acupuncture
www.acupuncture.com
www.medicalacupunture.com

Aromatherapy
www.naha.org

Callahan Technique
www.rogercallahan.com

Ayurvedic Medicine
www.ayurveda.com

Bioenergetic Bodywork
www.bioenergetic-therapy.com

Biological Dentistry
www.biologicaldentistry.org
www.holisticdental.org
www.hugginsappliedhealing.com

Bowen Therapy Technique
www.bowendirectory.com
www.boweninfo.com

Cancer
www.centurywellness.com

Candida Cleansing
www.candidaplan.com

Chelation Therapy
www.angelmedcenter.com/chelationtherapy
www.centurywellness.com

Chiropractic
www.chiropractic.org
www.americanchiropractic.org

Colon Therapy
www.i-act.org

Craniosacral Therapy
www.upledger.com

Detoxification and Cleansing
www.wecarespa.com
www.hippocratesinst.com

Energetic Rebalancing
www.aimprogram.com

Feldenkrais
www.feldenkrais.com

Hakomi
www.hakomiinstitute.com

Healing Touch
www.healingtouch.net

Heller Work
www.hellerwork.com

Herbal Medicine
www.herbalgram.org
www.ahpa.org

Homeopathic Medicine
www.homeopathyusa.org
www.homeopathic.org
www.homeopathy.org

Iridology
www.iridologyassn.org

Kinesiology
www.uskinesiologyinstitute.com
www.icak.com

Magnetic Field Therapy
www.polarpowermagnets.com

Massage Therapy
www.abmp.com
www.amtamassage.org
www.aobta.org

Music Therapy
www.musictherapy.org

Naturopathic Doctors
www.naturopathic.org
www.calnd.org
www.findnd.com
www.hanp.net

Neuro-Emotional Technique
www.NetMindBody.com

Organic Information
www.organic-center.org
www.organicconsumers.org
www.ota.com

Orthomolecular Medicine
www.orthomed.org

Osteopathic Medicine
www.academyofosteopathy.org
www.holisticmedicine.org
www.cranialacademy.com

Reflexology
www.reflexology-usa.net

Reiki
www.reiki.org

Rolfing
www.rolf.org

Rosen Method
www.rosenmethod.com

Sound Therapy
www.soundlistening.com

Sunlight Therapy
www.solarhealing.com
www.sungazing.com

Total Integration Therapy
www.touch4health.com

Organic/Kosher Meats
www.kolfoods.com

Trager Approach
www.trager.com

Other Helpful Websites:

www.dreammoods.com
www.drrathresearch.com
www.themeatrix.com
www.eatwellguide.com
www.davidwolfe.com
www.sunfood.net
www.mercola.com
www.thetruthaboutsplenda.com
www.healthfreedom.net

www.naturalcuresbook.com
www.whatthebleep.com
www.thesecret.tv
www.thecorporation.com
www.corporatewatch.org
www.prwatch.org
www.tvnewslies.org
www.foxbghsuit.com

Books:

I call this my Still Not Convinced? recommended reading list.

1. Not convinced that pasteurized and homogenized milk is deadly? Then read:
   - *Homogenized Milk May Cause Your Heart Attack: The XO Factor by Kurt A. Oster, M.D.*
   - *Don't Drink Your Milk! by Frank A. Oski, M.D.*
   - *Milk-The Deadly Poison by Robert Cohen*

2. Not Convinced That Aspartame (Nutrasweet®) And Monosodium Glutamate (MSG) Are Deadly? Then Read:
   - *Aspartame (NutraSweet®) Is It Safe? by H. J. Roberts, M.D.*
   - *Excitotoxins-The Taste that Kills by Russell L. Blaylock, M.D.*
   - *In Bad Taste: The MSG Symptom Complex by George R. Schwartz, M.D.*

3. Not convinced that you have a candida yeast overgrowth causing all types of medical problems including excess

weight, arthritis, depression, pms, acne, migraines, stress, constipation, bloating, skin rashes and more? Then read:

- *Lifeforce by Jeffrey S. McCombs, D.C.*

4. Not convinced that subtle energy therapies can cure virtually all disease? Then read:

- *Sanctuary by Stephen Lewis and Evan Slawson*
- *Vibrational Medicine by Richard Gerber, M.D.*
- *Energy Medicine-The Scientific Basis of Bioenergy Therapies by James L. Oschman and Candace Pert, Ph.D.*

5. Not convinced that food additives are a leading cause of illness? Then read:

- *Hard to Swallow by Doris Sarjeant and Karen Evans*

6. Not convinced the food industry is purposely creating foods that make you physically addicted, increase your appetite, make you fat and give you disease? Then read:

- *Fast Food Nation-The Dark Side of the All-American Meal by Eric Schlosser*
- *The Crazy Makers by Carol Simontacchi*
- *Genetically Engineered Food-Changing the Nature of Nature by Martin Teitel, Ph.D. and Kimberly A. Wilson*
- *Food Politics by Marion Nestle and Michael Pollan*
- *Restaurant Confidential: The Shocking Truth About what You're Really Eating When You're Eating Out by Michael F. Jacobson, Ph.D.*
- *Fat Land by Greg Critser*

7. Not convinced that vaccines are deadly, cause disease and should not be used? Then read:

- *A Shot in the Dark by Harris L. Coulter and Barbara Loe Fisher*
- *Vaccines: Are They Really Safe & Effective? by Neil Z. Miller*
- *What Your Doctor May Not Tell You About Children's Vaccinations by Stephanie Cave, M.D., F.A.A.F.P., with Deborah Mitchell*

8. Not convinced that cancer can be cured without drugs and surgery? Then read:
   - *The Cancer Cure That Worked! Fifty Years of Suppression by Barry Lynes*
   - *The Cancer Conspiracy by Barry Lynes*
   - *How to Fight Cancer & Win by William L. Fisher*
   - *The Breuss Cancer Cure by Rudolf Breuss*
   - *The Cancer Industry by Ralph W. Moss, Ph.D.*
   - *The Cure for All Cancers by Hulda Regehr Clark, Ph.D., N.D.*
   - *The Healing of Cancer-The Cures-the Cover-ups and the Solution Now by Barry Lynes*

9. Not convinced that your thoughts can make you sick or heal you? Then read:
   - *Anatomy of an Illness as Perceived by the Patient by Norman Cousins*
   - *Head First-The Biology of Hope and Healing Power of the Human Spirit by Norman Cousins*

10. Not convinced that you should never eat meat or poultry that is not organic? Then read:
    - *Slaughterhouse by Gail A. Eisnitz*
    - *No More Bull!: The Mad Cowboy Targets America's Worst Enemy: Our Food by Howard F. Lyman with Glen Merzer*
    - *Prisoned Chickens, Poisoned Eggs by Karen Davis, Ph.D.*

11. Not convinced that our food is loaded with chemicals causing illness and disease? Then read:
    - *The Chemical Feast by James S. Turner*
    - *A Chemical Feast by W. Harding Le Riche*
    - *Sowing the Wind by Harrison Wellford*

12. Not convinced that electromagnetic pollution is bombarding your body, causing all kinds of medical problems? Then read:

- *Cross Currents-The Promise of Electromedicine by Robert O. Becker, M.D.*

- *Electromagnetic Fields by B. Blake Levitt*

13. Not convinced that we all have an energetic field around us that is adversely affected by magnetic pollution? Then read:

- *The Unseen Self, Revised: Kirlian Photography Explained by Brian Snellgrove*

- *Kirlian Photography-A Hands-On Guide by John Iovine*

14. Not convinced that drugs are poisons and cause most disease? Then read:

- *Over Dose: The Case Against the Drug Companies Prescription Drugs, Side Effects, and Your Health by Jay S. Cohen, M.D.*

- *Bitter Pills: Inside the Hazardous World of Legal Drugs by Stephen Fried*

15. Not convinced that the pharmaceutical industry is purposely selling ineffective dangerous drugs, and working tirelessly to suppress natural, effective cures for disease? Then read:

- *Racketeering in Medicine-The Suppression of Alternatives by James P. Cater, M.D., Ph.D.*

- *The Drug Lords: America's Pharmaceutical Cartel by Tonda R. Bian*

- *The Big Fix by Katharine Greider*

- *The Assault on Medical Freedom by P. Joseph Lisa*

- *Disease-Mongers: How Doctors, Drug Companies, and Insurers Are Making You Feel Sick by Lynn Payer*

- *Under the Influence of Modern Medicine by Terry A. Rondberg, D.C.*

- *The Social Transformation of American Medicine by Paul Starr*

- *Medical Blunders: Amazing True Stories of Mad, Bad and Dangerous Doctors by Robert Youngson and Ian Schott*

16. Not convinced that psychiatry, and all psychiatric drugs harm patients and actually cause depression, suicide, violent acts, and disease? Then read:

- *Psychiatry: The Ultimate Betrayal by Bruce Wiseman*
- *Your Drug May Be Your Problem by Peter R. Breggin, M.D. and David Cohen*
- *Talking Back To Ritalin by Peter R. Breggin, M.D. and Dick Scruggs*
- *Talking Back To Prozac by Peter R. Breggin, M.D. and Ginger Ross*
- *The Antidepressant Fact Book by Peter R. Breggin, M.D.*
- *The Myth of Mental Illness by Thomas S. Szasz, M.D.*
- *The Manufacture of Madness by Thomas S. Szasz, M.D.*
- *Mad in America by Robert Whitaker*

17. Not convinced that calcium is a nutrient that most people are depleted in? Then read:

- *The Calcium Factor: The Scientific Secret of Health and Youth by Robert R. Barefoot and Carl J. Reich, M.D.*

18. Not convinced that if your body pH is alkaline you can virtually never get sick? Then read:

- *Alkalize or Die by Theodore A. Baroody*
- *Dynamic Health by Dr. M. Ted Morter, Jr.*
- *The Acid-Alkaline Diet for Optimum Health by Christopher Vasey and John Graham*
- *The pH Miracle by Robert O. Young, Ph.D. and Shelly Redford Young*

19. Not convinced that magnets can heal, alleviate pain, and cure disease? Then read:

- *Magnet Therapy: Discover the Powerful New Force in Health and Recovery by Gloria Vergari and Tony Cowell*
- *Healing with Magnets by Gary Null, Ph.D. with Vickie Riba Koestler*

20. Not convinced that aids is one of the greatest hoaxes and deceptions perpetrated on the american public? Then read:

- *Inventing the AIDS Virus by Peter H. Duesberg, Ph.D.*
- *AIDS: What the Government Isn't Telling You by Lorraine Day*
- *Infectious AIDS: Have We Been Misled? by Peter H. Duesberg, Ph.D.*
- *The AIDS War by John Lauritsen*
- *Do Insects Transmit AIDS? by Lawrence Miike*
- *Why We Will Never Win the War on AIDS by Bryan J. Ellison and Peter H. Duesberg, Ph.D.*

21. Not convinced that your digestive system is dysfunctional if you live in america? Then read:

- *Restoring Your Digestive Health by Jordan S. Rubin, N.M.D. and Joseph Brasco, M.D.*

22. Not convinced that stress, anxiety, and emotional problems can be cured almost instanty? Then read:

- *7 Steps to Overcoming Depression and Anxiety by Gary Null, Ph.D.*
- *Dianetics by L. Ron Hubbard.*

23. Not convinced that pain in any part of your body can be eliminated easily without drugs or surgery? Then read:

- *Pain Free: An Evolutionary Method for Stopping Chronic Pain by Peter Egoscue*
- *Instant Relief: Tell Me Where it Hurts and I'll Tell You What to Do by Peggy W. Brill, P.T. and Susan Suffes*
- *Pain Free at Your PC by Peter Egoscue*
- *Natural Relief from Aches & Pains by C. J. Puotinen*

24. Not convinced that women are being exploited by the medical establishment? Then read:

- *The Politics of Stupid by Susan Powter*
- *Hormone Replacement Therapy: Yes or No? by Betty Kamen, Ph.D.*

- *Alternative Medicine Guide to Women's Health by Burton Goldberg*
- *Male Practice: How Doctors Manipulate Women by Robert S. Mendelsohn, M.D.*

25. Not convinced that tap water containing fluoride, chlorine and other contaminants is a major cause of illness and disease? Then read:
    - *Fluoride: The Aging Factor by John Yiamouyannis, Ph.D.*
    - *Your Body's Many Cries for Water by F. Batmanghelidj, M.D.*
    - *Don't Drink the Water by Lono Kahuna Kupua A'o*
    - *Water-The Foundation of Youth, Health, and Beauty by William D. Holloway, Jr. and Herb Joiner-Bey, N.D.*
    - *The Water We Drink by Joshua L. Barzilay, M.D., Winkler G. Weinberg, M.D., and J. William Eley, M.D.*
    - *The Drinking Water Book by Colin Ingram*
    - *Water: For Health, For Healing, For Life by F. Batmanghelidj, M.D.*
    - *Water Wasteland by David Zwick with Marcy Benstock*

26. Not convinced that arthritis can be eliminated without drugs or surgery? Then read:
    - *Arthritis Defeated at Last! The Real Arthritis Cure by Len Sands, N.D., Ph.D., ACRP*
    - *Arthritis Beaten Today! by Len Sands, N.D., Ph.D., ACRP*

27. Not convinced that rebounding exercises strengthen every cell in the body, and lead to vibrant health and weight loss? Then read:
    - *Looking Good, Feeling Great by Karol Kuhn Truman and Alan Parkinson*
    - *Rebounding to Better Health by Linda Brooks*
    - *Urban Rebounding: An Exercise for the New Millennium by J. B. Berns*
    - *Harry and Sarah Sneider's Olympic Trainer by Harry and Sarah Sneider*

28. Not convinced that the FDA Is purposely suppressing natural cures for diseases and allows drug manufacturers to sell ineffective and dangerous drugs? Then read:

- *Innocent Casualties: The FDA's War Against Humanity by Elaine Feuer*
- *Stop the FDA: Save Your Health Freedom by John Mogenthaler and Steven W. Fowkes*
- *Hazardous to Our Health? by Robert Higgs*
- *Protecting America's Health: The FDA, Business and One Hundred Years of Regulation by Philip J. Hilts*

29. Not convinced that using oxygen can reverse aging, speed healing, and potentially cure many diseases? Then read:

- *Flood Your Body with Oxygen by Ed McCabe*
- *Stop Aging or Slow the Process: How Exercise With Oxygen Therapy (EWOT) Can Help by William Campbell Douglass II, M.D.*
- *Oxygen Healing Therapies by Nathaniel Altman*

30. Not convinced that yoga has amazing health benefits? Then read:

- *Ancient Secret of The Fountain of Youth by Peter Kelder and Bernie S. Siegel*
- *Bikram's Beginning Yoga Class by Bikram Choudhury with Bonnie Jones Reynolds*
- *Power Yoga by Beryl Bender Birch*

31. Not convinced that you can eliminate phobias, traumas, addictions and compulsions in as little as five minutes? Then read:

- *Tapping the Healer Within by Roger J. Callahan, Ph.D. with Richard Trubo*
- *Next Generation Herbal Medicine by Daniel B. Mowrey, Ph.D.*
- *Herbal Tonic Therapies by Daniel B. Mowrey, Ph.D.*

- *Prescription for Herbal Healing: An Easy to Use A-Z Reference by Phyllis A. Balch*

32. Not convinced that homeopathic medicines are a safe natural alternative to drugs and surgery and can cure disease and keep you healthy? Then read:

    - *Everybody's Guide to Homeopathic Medicines by Stephen Cummings, M.D. and Dana Ullman, M.P.H.*
    - *The Complete Homeopathy Handbook by Miranda Castro*

33. Not convinced that fibromyalgia can be eliminated naturally? Then read:

    - *The Fibromyalgia Relief Handbook by Chet Cunningham*

34. Not convinced that there are natural remedies for virtually every disease? Then read:

    - *The Cure for All Diseases by Hulda Reghr Clark, Ph.D., N.D.*
    - *Encyclopedia of Natural Medicine by Michael Murray, N.D. and Joseph Pizzorno, N.D.*
    - *Health and Nutrition Secrets That Can Save Your Life by Russell L. Blaylock, M.D.*
    - *The Natural Physician's Healing Therapies: Proven Remedies That Medical Doctors Don't Know About by Mark Stengler, N.D.*
    - *Alternative Medicine: The Definitive Guide by Larry Trivieri and Burton Goldberg*
    - *Dr. Duarte's The Most Common Diseases & Their Alternative Natural Therapies by Alex Duarte, O.D., Ph.D.*

35. Not convinced that you never have to get sick? Then read:

    - *You Can Be...Well At Any Age: Your Definitive Guide to Vibrant Health & Longevity by K. Steven Whiting, Ph.D.*
    - *How to Get Well: Dr. Airola's Handbook of Natural Healing by Paavo Airola, Ph.D.*
    - *Death by Diet: The Relation Between Nutrient Deficiency and Disease by Robert R. Barefoot*
    - *The Food Revolution by John Robbins and Dean Ornish*

36. Not convinced that proper deep breathing is one of the most beneficial things you can do? Then read:

- *Super Power Breathing for Super Energy, High Health & Longevity* by Paul C. Bragg, N.D. and Patricia Bragg, N.D., Ph.D.

37. Not convinced that your liver is clogged and needs cleansing? Then read:

- *The Liver Cleansing Diet* by Dr. Sandra Cabot, M.D.
- *The Amazing Liver and Gallbladder Flush* by Andreas Moritz
- *The Healthy Liver & Bowel Book* by Dr. Sandra Cabot, M.D.

38. Not convinced that there is an all natural cure for diabetes, and that the pharmaceutical industry offered $30 million to take it off the market? Then read:

- *The Natural Solution To Diabetes* by Richard Laliberte, Pat Harper and William Petit

39. Not convinced that juicing is absolutely needed if you want to get the nutrition your body needs? Then read:

- *The Juice Lady's Juicing For High-Level Wellness and Vibrant Good Looks* by Cherie Calbom, M.S.
- *The Juice Lady's Guide to Juicing for Health* by Cherie Calbom, M.S.
- *The Ultimate Smoothie Book* by Cherie Calbom, M.S.
- *The Joy of Juicing* by Gary Null, Ph.D.
- *Power Juices Super Drinks* by Steve Meyerowitz

40. Not convinced juice fasting is the most effective way to lose weight, cleanse the body of impurities, increase energy, and stimulate the immune system? Then read:

- *Juice Fasting & Detoxification* by Steve Meyerowitz
- *The Miracle of Fasting* by Paul C. Bragg, N.D. and Patricia Bragg, N.D., Ph.D.

41. Not convinced that colon cleansing is absolutely needed by every single person, and that doing so can alleviate illness and disease, increase metabolism and potentially slow or reverse aging? Then read:

- *Cleanse & Purify Thyself. Book One: The Cleanse by Richard Anderson, N.D., N.M.D.*
- *The Detox Diet: Third Edition by Elson M. Haas, M.D. and Daniella Chace*
- *How to Cleanse and Detoxify Your Body Today! by Elson M. Haas, M.D.*
- *Internal Cleansing by Linda Berry, D.C., C.C.N.*
- *The Master Cleanser by Stanley Burroughs*
- *Healthy Living: A Holistic Guide to Cleansing, Revitalization and Nutrition by Susana Lombardi*

42. Not convinced that toxins lodge in the fatty tissues of the body and are causing a host of physical and mental problems? Then read:

- *Clear Body, Clear Mind by L. Ron Hubbard*

43. Not convinced that proper diet can cure illness and lead to vibrant health and wellness? Then read:

- *The 7 Steps to Perfect Health by Gary Null, Ph.D.*
- *The Ultimate Healing System by Donald Lepore*
- *Diet for a New America by John Robbins*
- *Ultimate Lifetime Diet by Gary Null, Ph.D.*
- *Fell's Official Know-It-All Guide: Health & Wellness by Dr. M. Ted Morter, Jr.*

44. Not convinced that energy exists, and energy healing works? Then read:

- *The Healing Energy of Your Hands by Michael Bradford*
- *Quantum-Touch: The Power to Heal by Richard Gordon*
- *Wheels of Light: Chakras, Auras, and the Healing Energy of the Body by Rosalyn L. Bruyere*

45. Not convinced that hydrogenated oil and trans fats cause heart disease and a host of medical problems? Then read:
    * *Trans Fats by Judith Shaw*

46. Not convinced that watching too much television causes the body to become acidic, leading to disease? Then read:
    * *Four Arguments for the Elimination of Television by Jerry Mander*

47. Not convinced that lack of smiles, love and affection can cause illness and a host of emotional disorders? Then read:
    * *A Cry Unheard: New Insights Into The Medical Consequences of Loneliness by James Lynch*

48. Not convinced that what you say and how you say it have a powerful impact on your health and success? Then read:
    * *Should: How Habits of Language Shape Our Lives by Rebecca Smith*
    * *What You Say Is What You Get by Don Gossett*
    * *The Tongue: A Creative Force by Charles Capps*

49. Not convinced that writing things down causes them to happen? Then read:
    * *Write it Down, Make it Happen by Henriette Anne Klauser*

50. Not convinced that you can easily live to be over a hundred years old, never get sick, and that virtually everything i'm saying in this book is true? Then read:
    * *How Long Do You Choose to Live? A Question of a Lifetime by Peter Ragnar*
    * *Gary Null's Power Aging by Gary Null, Ph.D.*
    * *The 100 Simple Secrets of Healthy People by David Niven, Ph.D*
    * *Stopping the Clock by Ronald Klatz and Robert Goldman*
    * *The Longevity Strategy by David Mahoney and Richard Restak*
    * *Successful Aging by John W. Rowe, M.D. and Robert L.Kahn, Ph.D.*

- *The Okinawa Program by Bradley J. Willcox, M.D., Craig Willcox, Ph.D., and Makoto Suzuki, M.D.*
- *On My Own at 107: Reflections on Life Without Bessie by Sarah L. Delany with Amy Hill Hearth and Brian M. Kotsky*
- *Having Our Say: The Delany Sisters' First 100 Years by Sarah L. Delany and Elizabeth Delany with Amy Hill Hearth*
- *Living to 100 by Thomas T. Perls, M.D., M.P.H. and Margery Hutter Silver, Ed.D with John F. Lauerman*
- *Centenarians: The Bonus Years by Lynn Peters Alder, J.D.*
- *If I Live to be 100 by Neenah Ellis*
- *On Being 100 by Liane Enkelis*
- *Centenarians by Dale Richard Perelman*

51. Still not convinced that it's always all about the money, and corruption is permeating corporations and government in america and around the world? Then read:

- *The Informant: A True Story by Kurt Eichenwald*
- *Serpent on the Rock: Crime, Betrayal and the Terrible Secrets of Prudential Bache by Kurt Eichenwald*
- *Rats in the Grain: The Dirty Tricks and Trial of Archer Daniels Midland, the Supermarket to the World by James B. Leiber*
- *Funny Money by Mark Singer*

About the Author

KEVIN TRUDEAU is widely regarded as one of the nation's foremost consumer advocates. He's a New York Times bestselling author who has sold over thirty million books, including six million copies of the original *Natural Cures* book. Adopting as both his business and personal mission statement a vow to "positively impact the whole person," Kevin has built a global business empire that has marketed or sold products he personally uses and believes in 100 percent. Kevin knows from personal experience how big business and government try to debunk individuals who promote products that could hurt the profits of the giant multinational corporations. Kevin is also dedicated to the formation of various foundations to pursue these goals, and has donated part of his fortune for that purpose.